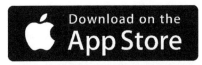
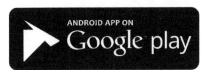

ISBN 978-1-5278-3957-1
PIBN 10123656

1 MONTH OF
FREE
READING

at

www.ForgottenBooks.com

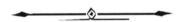

By purchasing this book you are eligible for one month membership to ForgottenBooks.com, giving you unlimited access to our entire collection of over 700,000 titles via our web site and mobile apps.

To claim your free month visit:
www.forgottenbooks.com/free123656

English
Français
Deutsche
Italiano
Español
Português

www.forgottenbooks.com

Mythology Photography **Fiction**
Fishing Christianity **Art** Cooking
Essays Buddhism Freemasonry
Medicine **Biology** Music **Ancient**
Egypt Evolution Carpentry Physics
Dance Geology **Mathematics** Fitness
Shakespeare **Folklore** Yoga Marketing
Confidence Immortality Biographies
Poetry **Psychology** Witchcraft
Electronics Chemistry History **Law**
Accounting **Philosophy** Anthropology
Alchemy Drama Quantum Mechanics
Atheism Sexual Health **Ancient History**
Entrepreneurship Languages Sport
Paleontology Needlework Islam
Metaphysics Investment Archaeology
Parenting Statistics Criminology
Motivational

Mary A. Stolz.

Mary A. Stolz.

iseases

OF THE

Digestive System

BY

E. O. ADAMS, M. D.

*Professor of the Theory and Practice of Medicine
and Clinical Medicine. The Cleveland
Homœopathic Medical College, Mem-
ber of the American Institute
of Homœopathy, etc.*

The Cleveland Homœopathic Publishing Co.
1910

1910

PREFACE.

IN no department of Internal Medicine have there been as many advances made during the last few years, as in that part pertaining to the digestive tract. These advances have resulted from knowledge obtained by recent physiological experiments, from increased surgery in these regions and from a development of laboratory methods for investigating the functional activities of these organs.

This book is designed:—

1 To give as accurately and concisely as possible the newer ideas which have developed, in addition to the older and established ones.

2. To give a technique for laboratory methods of diagnosis which is as simple and practical as is that used in examining the urine.

3. To give directions in regard to dietetics which are in accordance with modern knowledge of the chemistry of foods and of the physiology of digestion.

4. To give remedies, together with their indications which the experience of fifteen years of especial attention to this class of diseases has demonstrated to be of value.

The book is not intended to be encyclopaedic, but to be concise and practical.

E. O. ADAMS, M. D.

668 Rose Bldg., Cleveland, O.

TABLE OF CONTENTS.

PART I.—THE ŒSOPHAGUS.

PART II.—THE STOMACH.

PART III.—THE INTESTINE.

CONTENTS.

Part I — The Oesophagus.

CHAPTER I.

ŒSOPHAGITIS.

Etiology.—This may occur as an extension of inflammation from adjoining structures, as from the pharynx above or the stomach below. It may be caused by excessively hot or cold drinks or foods, or by chemical irritants, as the strong acids or alkalies. It may also be traumatic as a result of swallowing hard, sharp substances, or the introduction of instruments. In infants, it is sometimes seen as a result of nursing from unclean or sore nipples, or it may be from an extension of thrush. In exceptional cases it may be secondary to diphtheria or other infectious disease, or to constitutional diseases as tuberculosis, syphilis, anæmia or nephritis.

Pathology.—The same as of catarrhal processes elsewhere, and consists of a swollen, reddened, painful mucous membrane, covered by an excessive secretion of mucus. The pathology may extend no further than this, or may progress to a stage of ulceration. It is especially apt to do this when the exciting cause has been some irritant poison, or traumatism. If ulceration does develop, it results in a formation of scar tissue, which upon contracting produces more or less stenosis. In the case of strong acids or alkalies, this form of pathology may progress to such an extent that the lumen of the tube becomes entirely obliterated.

Symptomatology.—The principal symptom is pain on swallowing. Between the acts of swallowing there may be a dull soreness behind the sternum, possibly extending through to the back. Talking may produce pain, especially if the upper part of the œsophagus is affected. Sometimes the parts are so sensitive that attempts at swallowing cause a spasmodic contraction with ejection of the contents, which may possibly be streaked with blood. There is apt to be much thirst, which can only be relieved with difficulty because of the pain caused by swallowing. There is usually some fever, but this is not often high. If an ulcer forms, the symptoms, especially the pain, become intensified. Then, upon the development of the cicatricial tissue, with resulting stenosis, the dysphagia increases. A difficulty in swallowing food becomes marked, and if the condition becomes a severe one it may be impossible for either food or drink to reach the stomach.

Diagnosis.—If it is simply a case of catarrhal œsophagitis, a diagnosis can generally be made from the pain on swallowing, which is located below the pharynx or other portion of the throat. If an ulcer is present it can generally only be diagnosed positively by inspection through an œsophagoscope. If stricture develops, it can be determined by the difficulty of swallowing foods, while its extent and narrowness may be determined by passing œsophageal sounds or bougies of different sizes.

Prognosis.—Catarrhal œsophagitis usually recovers within a few days. If an ulcer forms, the condition, is more serious and may result fatally as a result of perforation or hæmorrhage. However, such outcomes are rare, but the stenosis following ulceration makes the case a long lasting one, with possibly never a complete recovery. The difficulty of taking sufficient food may cause malnutrition, or even starvation.

Treatment.—An important element of the treatment is rest to the part. If the attack is at all severe, feeding should be done by rectum, and nothing at all swallowed until a subsidence of the severity ensues. Then a careful resort to liquids and soft foods may be made. If the trouble has been caused by an irritant poison, of course, give the proper antidote as quickly as possible in order to reduce the damage to the minimum. The remedies most frequently useful, are:—

Aconite 3x.—In the early stage with fever, thirst, restlessness and anxiety. Pain extending to the back, worse on moving.

Arnica 6x.—When caused by traumatism, as swallowing a large or hard bolus, or injuries resulting from the passing of instruments. There are stinging, darting pains, or a feeling of soreness.

Belladonna 3x.—Severe pain, considerable fever, œsophageal spasm. There is much sensitiveness.

Cantharides 2x.—Especially useful when the inflammation has been caused by burns or scalds. There is marked dysphagia, with a feeling of burning and constriction.

Arsenicum alb. 3x.—Burning pain, soreness, dryness and constriction. All food is ejected. Pains cause shuddering and chilliness. Cramping pains with pressure behind the sternum. Restlessness and thirst.

Mercurius corr. 6x.—Burning and aching. Intensely dry feeling; deglutition difficult and causes an attack of suffocation. Fœtid breath. Apt to be an extension from stomatitis and to be accompanied with salivation. If ulceration with cicatrices and stenosis develops, the case becomes a surgical one, and will probably need to be treated by dilatation, or, possibly, a gastrostomy for the purpose of putting food directly into the stomach will have to be performed.

CHAPTER II.

FUNCTIONAL STENOSIS OF THE ŒSOPHAGUS.

Definition.—A difficulty or inability to make food pass through the entire extent of the œsophageal canal, even when no organic obstruction exists. The difficulty generally is found at the cardiac extremity.

Etiology.—The causes of such condition are not well understood. It is more frequent in people having an unstable nervous system, for instance hysteria. Sometimes it develops without such stigmata being present. Two theories have been proposed to explain the mechanism of the condition. The first one pre-supposes that in all cases there is a minute fissure at the opening into the stomach, and that the irritation of food endeavoring to pass this fissure results in spasmodic contraction to a sufficient extent to produce a partial or complete closure.

The other theory is based upon the claim that food is conducted through the œsophagus as a result of the action of five nerves. The upper four of these nerves acting in succession from above downward, cause a peristaltic movement which passes the bolus down the canal to the cardiac orifice.

That normally the fifth nerve then causes a relaxation of this orifice, permitting the food to drop into the stomach. In the condition under consideration, however, owing to some abnormality in this nerve or at the center from which it arises, it does not functionate, and so the orifice remains closed. It is impossible to say at present whether either of these theories is correct or not.

Symptomatology.—The symptoms generally appear during adult life, although it has been seen in childhood. Usually they come on gradually, difficulty in swallowing being the most prominent one. At first, this may apply only to solid food, but later even liquids are taken with difficulty or not at all. Frequently a part or the whole of a glass of milk, for instance, may be swallowed, followed by a sensation of fulness along the course of the œsophagus, until the entire amount is returned without having entered the stomach at all. This retention of the food above the seat of stricture causes distension and finally dilatation. In most cases there will be periods, possibly lasting only a few minutes, when there seemingly is some relaxation of the stricture, and it is at such times that food may be taken to support life. The patient acquires a habit of stretching the neck, pressing on the chest with the hands, and resorting to other means in an effort to force the food into the stomach. Often the action of these extraordinary muscles of deglutition will have but scant effect in accomplishing the desired end. Because of the inability to eat sufficient food, emaciation, anœmia and prostration develop.

Diagnosis.—The other affections from which this trouble will have to be differentiated, are cicatricial stenosis, new growths either of the œsophagus itself or external to it and pressing upon it, and diverticuli.

In cicatricial stenosis there is always a history of an ulcer, probably resulting from some irritant poison or from scalds.

The symptoms of a new growth, especially cancer of the œsophagus, may resemble this condition. But with cancer, as a rule, the symptoms are more stable and do not present periods of remission. There is also more pain of a burning, lancinating character, and the development of cachexia in addition to the anæmia resulting from insufficient nourishment. Growths of the mediastinum, aneurysm of the aorta, or other external enlargemen pressing upon the œsophagus will have to be considered, but like internal tumors their progress is generally more steady and other distinguishing symptoms will be present.

Cases have been reported of children being born with diverticuli leading off from the œsophagus. Such subjects also have trouble in swallowing, but these cases can generally be separated from the difficulty under consideration, by the facts that they are congenital and do not offer periods of partial remission. In some cases, filling the œsophagus with bismuth sub-nitrate suspended in a solution, and skiagraphing the area will assist in diagnosing the condition.

Prognosis.—This form of œsophageal stenosis is apt to be a long lasting trouble, especially if radical treatment is not resorted to. However, no reports of death directly due to it have been reported. Often the patients will reach a considerable degree of mal-nutrition, but still they always succeed in getting down enough food to support life.

Treatment.—The diet usually should be liquid, or at least soft, and given during the periods when some relaxation of the cardiac orifice exists. The patients generally soon learn when such periods are present, and can act accordingly. Improving the nerve tone by methods ordinarily resorted to, may modify to some extent the severity of the symptoms, especially in hysterical cases. Remedies, except for such purpose, are not of much use, although in one of my cases it seemed that food could be swallowed somewhat better immediately after taking a physiological dose of glonoin. A case has also been reported in which atropine, given in sufficient dose to cause relaxation of circular muscle fibres, has had the same effect.

However, the treatment is chiefly surgical. Probably the best method is by means of a properly shaped distensible bag on the end of a stomach tube. By careful manipulation this can generally be insinuated past the strictured point, and the bag may then be distended by water pressure by means of a syringe of sufficient strength. The stricture being thus forcibly dilated a few times, marked relief ensues. One must learn by experience as to the amount of dilatation needed, care being exercised that rupture or damage to the œsophagus is not produced.

CHAPTER III.

CANCER OF THE ŒSOPHAGUS.

This condition is comparatively rare, as in 2289 deaths from cancer, but 13 of them affected the œsophagus.

It may affect any part of the tube, though it is most frequent at the lower third. It is usually of the epitheliomatous variety, beginning in the mucous membrane, and extending to the other coats. It may entirely encircle the tube, then break down and ulcerate. As a result of this, perforation into the air passages or peritoneum may possibly occur.

Symptomatology.—There is a gradually increasing dysphagia, which may progress until swallowing is impossible. In the latter stages this may be somewhat relieved as a result of sloughing. Digestion is much impaired, and this fact together with the one that sufficient food cannot be swallowed, causes rapid emaciation and prostration. Pressure of the growth on the trachea may cause dyspnœa. There is much pain of a lancinating character extending through to the back, or downward to the stomach.

Diagnosis.—Cancer of the œsophagus may be suspected in an individual of the cancerous age, who presents a gradually advancing stenosis and sharp lancinating pains. The only way to convert this suspicion into a certainty is by microscopical examination of fragments which may be ejected with food, or by the passage of the œsophageal sound.

Prognosis.—Death always results, usually within a year.

Treatment.—Is only palliative. While food can yet pass, a nourishing diet should be given to keep up nutrition as well as possible. When food can no longer reach the stomach, the case becomes a surgical one. Then dilatation of the œsophagus, carefully performed may be of some avail; if not, gastrotomy, or an incision by which food may be put directly into the stomach, may be necessary.

Part II.—The Stomach.

CHAPTER I.

EXAMINATION OF THE STOMACH.

Before beginning the study of diseases of the stomach, it will be well to consider briefly some of the methods by which information of this organ and its functions may be obtained. Such methods may be classified under three divisions:—

1.—History.
2.—Physical examination.
3.—Examination with the stomach tube.

In securing the patient's story, the best results will be obtained if they are induced to commence at the beginning of the trouble; especially if it is one of long standing. Most patients are inclined to start in at once with their present symptoms, but it seems that the more many of them talk about these, the fainter becomes their remembrance of the incipient symptoms and the more inclined are they to modify the symptoms of their past, so that they will co-incide with those now present. Especially is this true of those whose digestive difficulties are of functional nature. Often by holding them at first to those abnormal sensations which they experienced possibly years ago, then gradually leading them up to the present time, a much clearer perspective of their condition will be obtained than if they had commenced with their present distress and gone backward.

The importance of a careful history will be more fully seen, when we take up consideration of the diseases of the

digestive organs, together with their complications and
sequelæ. One instance out of several may be mentioned,
where an inflammation, occurring sometime in the past,
has involved the stomach, duodenum, bile tract, appendix,
or other part. Although the inflammation has subsided yet
there remain cicatrices or adhesions which are now interfering with the proper performance of the digestive functions. Such symptoms might have been attributed to some
entirely different condition, unless the past history had
been carefully elicited and correctly interpreted.

The past health, as regards affections of organs other
than the digestive, should also be considered. For instance, affections of the heart, blood, kidneys, pelvic organs, nervous system,—in fact almost any organ of the
body, may manifest themselves by giving rise to imper-
fections of the digestive process. The one who under-
stands general diagnosis the best, will be the most successful in arriving at correct opinions in regard to diseases of
the gastro-intestinal tract.

When the consideration of the subjective symptoms is
reached, attention should be given to abnormal sensations,
as pain, fullness, pressure, burning, etc., to belching,
nausea or vomiting, the appetite, whether the distress is
aggravated or not by eating, the effects of different kinds
of foods, frequency and character of the stools, intestinal
tympanitis, and to anything else that might arise in individual cases.

PHYSICAL EXAMINATION.

In examining for troubles within the abdomen, it is generally best to have the patient in a recumbent position, the
head resting comfortably on a low pillow, and the knees
drawn up. Then ask the patient to relax the abdominal
muscles as much as possible. The methods of examination,

given in the order in which they are generally employed, are—Inspection, Succussion, Palpation, Percussion and Auscultation.

Inspection should begin by giving attention to the patient's general appearance as regards color of the skin and mucous membranes, state of nutrition, expressions of pain or suffering, presence or absence of neurotic stigmata and condition of the circulation. Then noting more especially the abdomen itself, see if there is distention by gas or ascites, if the contour is normal, or if there is an epigastric depression with prominence of the lower abdomen. In rare instances, a tumor may be large enough or so placed that it can be seen. Sometimes peristaltic movements may be so pronounced that they may be seen; especially may this be so in emaciated subjects.

Succussion is performed by gently tapping over the epigastric region with the tips of the fingers. In many cases it gives rise to a splashing sound which can be easily heard. This indicates that there is both air and fluid in the stomach. The importance of this sign is variously estimated by different authorities. Some claim that if a splashing is heard it always indicates that the gastric walls are not contracting on their contents as firmly as they should, and therefore that there is dilatation, or at least motor insufficiency. This seems too broad a statement to make, although in these conditions this splashing is certainly more often prominent. But it is sometimes heard in people with no other signs of digestive disturbances, and with no other signs of such troubles. Some have also claimed that by succussion the position of the greater curvature of the stomach can be determined. This is hardly true for two reasons. First, in tapping the abdomen even on a lower level than the margin of the stomach, the splashing is often heard. Secondly, it is practically impossible to differentiate between splashing occurring in the stomach, and that produced in the transverse colon. So about the only value of the sign is that, if it is heard at a time after eating or drinking when the stomach should be empty, it indicates dilatation, motor insufficiency or pyloric obstruction, with the result that food is stagnating in the stomach.

Palpation is the most valuable of these physical methods. To perform it properly, the patient's muscles must be as flaccid as possible, and the stomach and intestines well emptied. The examiner's hands should be warm, and contact be made with the palmar surface of the flattened hand and fingers. By this method, tumors may sometimes be felt, the size and position of the stomach determined to a certain extent and the presence of sore spots or general tenderness be determined. In addition, many times the condition of neighboring organs may be determined, as for instance, enlargement or tumor of the liver, gall stones, sometimes tumor of the pancreas, abnormal motility or size of the kidneys, tumors of the omentum, and tumor or masses of impacted fæces in the intestine.

Percussion may be of value in detecting dullness of suspected tumors, in differentiating between tumors of the stomach and those of other organs, and to some extent in determining the size and position of the stomach. This latter is difficult to do with any degree of exactness, because the upper part of the viscus is covered by the left lobe of the liver, while the lower part is resting on the transverse colon, and can scarcely be distinguished from it. Much assistance is secured in employing this method, by distending the stomach with gas or air. This may be done by giving nearly a teaspoonful of bi-carbonate of soda in half a glass of water, followed by the same amount of tartaric acid. Or, if the patient is accustomed to the stomach tube, it is better to pass this instrument and pump air into the stomach by means of an atomizer bulb. In this way the amount of dilatation of the stomach can be exactly gauged. After employing one of these means, one can more nearly outline the stomach and determine its size and position. It will also sometimes help to locate a tumor, and if this be present determine whether it is of the stomach or elsewhere.

Auscultation has but a limited use in examining the stomach. It has been employed with some success in conjunction with percussion, to more exactly distinguish between the different sounds. It may also be used in cases of suspected stenosis of the cardiac orifice. The method is to have the patient drink a glass of water. Normally in from six to twelve seconds the sound of the water entering the stomach may be heard. If this is absent or delayed, it indicates some form of obstruction in the œsophagus.

The same as in taking the patient's history, physical methods of diagnosis should also be employed outside of the gastro-intestinal tract. Heart, lung, liver, kidney, blood, nerve, genito urinary, toxic and many other diseases may, and often do have a pronounced effect in causing digestive troubles. Frequently, serious diseases of other parts will so affect digestion that the patient will complain only of such troubles. Therefore if one confines himself to seat of greatest distress only, he will often be led astray diagnostically and therapeutically.

EXAMINATION WITH THE STOMACH TUBE.

Laboratory methods which are used in connection with the stomach, are employed for the purpose of gaining information as regards,—

1.—The secretory function.

2.—The absorptive function.

3.—The motor function.

4.—The size of the stomach.

5.—The discovery of adventitious substances in the stomach contents.

In making an examination for the purpose of studying the secretory function, it is customary to have the patient prepare by eating a test meal. Then a certain length of time afterwards,—the length of time depending on the character of the meal,—the stomach is emptied by means of a soft-rubber stomach tube. This can generally be done without difficulty if an effort is first made to gain the patient's confidence. It is best to instruct him to push the head forward,—instead of backward as is the natural inclination. To open the mouth widely,—first removing any teeth on plates, if present. Then directing the tube backward, possibly tilting it downward if the tongue will permit, ask the patient to swallow. This attempt at swallowing will first cause the pharyngeal muscles to grasp the tube, and then as they relax it may be pushed downward till the stomach is reached, in the average individual, a distance of sixteen inches from the line of the teeth. As the cavity of the stomach is reached, in the majority of cases, attempts at retching usually cause the contents to come up through the tube and they may be caught in some receptacle for that purpose. If they do not come at once, the patient should be told to strain as if making an effort to pass stool. Or, instead of thus forcing evacuation, the contents of the stomach may be aspirated by means of a large rubber bulb, which, being attached to the extremity of the tube, is first compressed and then grad-
ꝟ allowed to expand. When the contents are received,

they may be examined microscopically for bacteria, blood, pus, epithelium, shreds of tissue, meat fibres, etc., or to determine the stage of digestion of the starch cells.

The test meal most frequently used is called the Ewald test breakfast. This consists of a roll and a glass of water, or a cup of tea without milk or sugar. The time for withdrawal is one hour after eating. Leube's test dinner is sometimes used. This consists of 400 c. c. of soup, a portion of beefsteak or roast beef, some potatoes and a slice of bread. The time for withdrawal is four hours after the meal. Boas' test breakfast is useful when we desire to remove the possibility of taking something which might introduce into the stomach any lactic acid forming material. This breakfast consists of oat meal soup prepared by adding one tablespoonful of oat meal to a quart of water and boiling it until there is but a pint remaining.

The stomach contents should be filtered before making the chemical examination. In analyzing they may be subjected to the following tests:—

1.—Reaction.
2.—Free hydrochloric acid.
3.—Total acidity.
4.—Rennin.
5.—Pepsin.
6.—Pro-peptone.
7.—Peptones.
8.—Proteolytic power.
9.—Dextrin.
10.—Erythrodextrin.
11.—Achroodextrin.
12.—Maltose.
13.—Amylolytic power.
14.—Lactic acid.
15.—Other organic acids.
16.—Bile.

Reaction:—This may be taken by litmus paper, in the same manner as in the urine. Normally it is acid.

Free Hydrochloric Acid:—Qualitatively its presence may be determined by Congo paper. This paper is red, and turns to dark blue or purple in the presence of this acid.

However in order to be of practical benefit it is necessary to make a quanitative examination, and the method usually employed is the so-called,—

Toepfer's Test:—To perform this test two re-agents are needed.—1.—A 0.5 per cent. alcoholic solution of di-methyl-amido-azo-benzol. 2.—A deci-normal sodium hydrate solution. This consists of four grammes of pure, crystallized sodium hydrate dissolved in 1000 c. c. of distilled water. But as sodium hydrate is a very unstable article, it is necessary to employ certain precautions in order to get a correct solution. The best way is as follows:—Dissolve 4 grammes of sodium hydrate, as pure as can be obtained, in 900 c. c. of water. Then dissolve one-tenth gramme of dry oxalic acid crystals in 10 c. c. of distilled water, and add two or three drops of a one per cent. alcoholic solution of phenolthallein, as an indicator. From a graduated burette the sodium hydrate solution is then added to the oxalic acid solution, until a scarlet color appears. This should require 15.9 c. c. of the sodium solution. But as this was purposely made too strong, less than this will be used. To find the amount of water necessary to add in order to make it of the proper strength, employ the following computation. Let C represent the number of c. c. of water which must be added to the remainder of the 900 c. c. Let N represent the number of the 900 c. c. remaining after the titration. Let d represent the difference between 15.9 c. c. the number theoretically required, and the number which actually were used in the titration, and let n represent the number of c. c. which were employed. The formula $C = \frac{Nd}{n}$ worked out, will give the number of c. c. of water which must be added to the sodium solution to make it correct. After this water has been added.

it is better to make a second titration in exactly the same way, with the corrected solution, to see that it is exact.

Toepfer's test consists in finding the number of c. c. of this deci-normal sodium hydrate solution required to neutralize all the free hydrochloric acid in 100 c. c. of the filtered stomach contents. Take 5 c. c. of the gastric filtrate, and add two or three drops of the di-methyl-amido-azo-benzol solution. In the presence of free hydrochloric acid this gives a bright red color. From a graduated burette add carefully, drop by drop, the deci-normal solution until the red color disappears and a turbid yellow color is produced. At this point read from the burette the number of c. c. used, and multiply this by twenty, because only 5 c. c. of the stomach contents were used instead of 100 c. c. The result is spoken of as the degree of free hydrochloric acid. As example, suppose that 1.4 c. c. of the sodium solution were used to destroy the red color in 5 c. c. of the filtered contents. Then multiply 1.4 by 20 which equals 28.0. In such a case the degree of free hydrochloric acid is spoken of as 28. If the secretions of the stomach are normal, the degree should be between 20 and 30. In some cases of hypochlorhydria it may be much below 20 or even be entirely absent. On the other hand, in cases of hyperchlorhydria it may reach a degree of 40, 50, or even up to 100.

The total acidity includes all acids present; that is, the free acid, that part of it which has combined with the proteid elements of the food, and any organic acids which may be present. To make a quantative test for total acidity, two re-agents are required.—

1.—A 1 per cent. alcoholic solution of phenolthallein as indicator.

2.—The deci-normal sodium hydrate solution.

To 5 c. c. of the filtered stomach contents, two or three drops of the phenolthallein solution are added. This gives a turbid yellow color. To this, from a graduated burette, the sodium solution is added until a bright red color results. The number of c. c. used, multiplied by 20 gives the degree of total acidity. Example, suppose 2.6 c. c. of the deci-normal solution were added. This multiplied by 20 equals 52.0. Then the degree of total acidity is spoken of as being 52. The normal degree is from 40 to 60.

Rennin:—To 10 c. c. of fresh cow's milk, add a few drops of the filtrate which has been exactly neutralized by the sodium hydrate solution. Mix and keep at a temperature of about 100 degrees Fahrenheit. If rennin is present, the milk should be curdled in 10 minutes.

Pepsin:—A thin disk of hard boiled egg albumin is put in 10 c. c. of the filtrate. If free hydrochloric acid is not present, add 5 drops of the commercial dilute acid. If pepsin is present to the normal amount, the egg albumin will be dissolved in three or four hours.

Pro-peptone:—This represents the intermediate stage in the digestion of the proteid elements of the food into peptones. Their presence may be determined by uniting an equal amount of the filtrate and a saturated solution of sodium chloride. If they are in normal amount, a white precipitate will form.

Peptones:—First precipitate the pro-peptones by the test given above, and filter them out. Make this filtrate alkaline by adding sodium hydrate solution; add a few drops of a 1 per cent. solution of copper sulphate. If peptones are present, as they should be, a purplish or violet color will be produced.

Pro-teolytic Power:—This may be determined by means of Mett's test. Suck fluid egg albumin into a glass tube

1 to 2 m. m. in diameter, and raise it to a temperature of 95 degrees Centigrade for the purpose of coagulating the albumin. The tube is then cut into short pieces. One of these pieces is put into some gastric filtrate and kept at a temperature of 37 to 38 degrees Centigrade. After a definite length of time, the column of egg albumin which has been digested is read by means of a millimetre scale and a microscope of low magnifying power. In employing this test, it has been shown by experiments that the quantity of pepsin in fluids is proportionate to the square of the rapidity of digestion, i. e., the square of the length of the column expressed in m. m. Thus in comparing two samples of gastric filtrate, if one digests a column of 2 m. m., and the other 3 m. m., the relative strength of the proteolytic power is 4 and 9.

Dextrin, Erythrodextrin and Achroodextrin:—These starchy derivatives may be determined by means of an iodine solution, of just sufficient strength to be a light yellow. Put two or three drops of the tincture of iodine in 10 c. c. of distilled water. Then add a few drops of the gastric filtrate. If dextrin is present, the solution turns blue; if erythrodextrin, it turns red; if achroodextrin, it turns white. Dextrin is simply cooked starch, and should be absent from the stomach contents, because the ptyalin of the saliva should have changed it to one of the later starchy derivatives. Erythrodextrin is the first stage of such digestion and a small amount of this is usually present in a healthy stomach. Achroodextrin is the next stage, and it should be present in rather a larger degree.

Maltose:—Is the end product in the process of starch digestion, and should be present to a considerable degree one hour after a test breakfast. It may be detected in the gastric filtrate, by Fehling's or Trommer's tests, the same as in urine.

Amylolytic Power:—This is simply determining the digestive power of ptyalin in the saliva, and is done in exactly the same way as in testing for the proteolytic power of the pepsin, except that a colored starch paste is used instead of the egg albumin.

Lactic Acid:—The presence of this acid may be determined by Uffelmann's test. To 10 c. c. of water in a test tube, add two or three drops of carbolic acid and the same amount of ferric chloride. This gives an amethyst blue color. To this, add a few drops of the gastric filtrate. If lactic acid is present, a yellow, canary color results. When this acid is present in sufficient amount to respond to this test, it indicates a considerable degree of lactic acid fermentation taking place in the stomach, greater than is apt to occur unless there is a pyloric obstruction of sufficient degree to cause a marked stagnation of the chyme. In ulcerative or cicatricial stenosis, there is usually present a sufficient degree of hydrochloric acid to prevent such a marked fermentation. Therefore, the only form of pyloric stenosis apt to give rise to this condition is carcinomatous, in which, as a rule, there is absence of free hydrochloric acid. Therefore the finding of lactic acid is strongly suggestive of cancer of the pylorus. However, it must not be considered an absolutely pathognomonic sign, for occasionally a case will be seen where this acid is present in small amounts, and still there is no cancer. In a somewhat larger number of cases, the acid will not be found when cancer is present, especially in the earlier stages of those cancers developing upon the base of an old ulcer.

Other Organic Acids:—Acetic, butyric and succinic acids are sometimes present in stomach contents. They indicate some stagnation, such as perhaps may be found in certain cases of motor insufficiency. To detect them, make an ethereal extract of the stomach contents by shaking one c. c. of the filtrate with four c. c. of ether, and allow them to separate. Carefully, by means of a pipette, allow some of this ethereal filtrate to trickle down the side of a test tube in which there are a few c. c. of distilled water with just enough ferric chloride in it to cause the slightest appreciable tinge. If acetic acid is present there will be a rusty red ring at the point of junction of the two fluids. Succinic acid gives a dark mahogany ring, butyric acid an orange ring.

CONSIDERATIONS IN REGARD TO ANALYSIS OF STOMACH CONTENTS.

In order to profit by analysis of gastric contents, it is necessary to give attention to certain points. The amount of secretion, as well as its degree of acidity and proteolytic power, varies considerably, depending upon the variety of food eaten, the length of time elapsing after taking food, and the mental attitude of the patient during and after eating. Therefore, in order to have a good understanding of the patient's gastric secretions, it is necessary to make a number of analyses, at different times after eating, using different test meals, and endeavoring to acquire the patient's confidence and ease of mind. For, if a patient has eaten a first test meal, with expectation perhaps of appearing before a strange doctor and having a stomach tube passed,—which performance may have been described by friends as being extremely unpleasant,—the peptic glands, —controlled entirely as they are by nerves from both the cerebro-spinal and sympathetic nervous systems,—will give forth a much different secretion, than they will during the every day life of the same individual.

In order to study more in detail features which influence the gastric secretion, as well as to have in condensed form a table which can be referred to when considering the therapeutics, especially the physiological therapeutics of functional abnormalities of secretion, we suggest the following classification of those agents, which by physiological experiment have been proven either to increase or to decrease gastric secretion, or to influence the quantity or quality of the gastric ferments. Undoubtedly there are other agents which have such effects, but these are the only ones proven.

1.—Agents which increase gastric secretion:
    a.—A good appetite.
    b.—Meat extracts.
    c.—Mental ease and comfort.
    d.—Water.
    e.—Bitters.
    f.—Tart foods.

2.—Agents which decrease gastric secretion:
    a.—Lack of appetite.
    b.—Oil.
    c.—Mucus producing agents.
    d.—Alkalies.
    e.—Pain.

As a stimulant to gastric secretion, a good appetite is of chief value. It has been shown both by experiments on dogs, and clinically in man by analysis of the stomach contents, that if there is no appetite because of recent eating, illness or anything else, gastric secretion will not be stimulated by food nearly as much as when a considerable degree of hunger, with a relish for the food, is present. This fact should be considered in analyzing stomach contents and may also be used in treatment.

Although all foods presenting proteids stimulate peptic secretion, it has been proven that the meat extracts are more powerful in this direction than anything else. These may be secured by eating the meat itself, or from bouillon, soups, etc., made from meat. Liebig's beef extract acts very energetically in this manner. Therefore, where a decreased secretion is present, beginning a meal with bouillon made from some such extract is proper. However, after secretion has started, the digestive power of gastric juice secreted after eating meat is not as great as that secreted after eating bread. Experiments on dogs have shown that the juice secreted after eating bread has a digestive power of 44, after meat 16, and after milk 11. Whereas the acidity varies thus: Meat 0.56%, bread 0.46%.

The psychical condition has much to do with gastric secretion. If one is feeling perfectly at ease mentally, possibly enjoying social intercourse, with all the adjuncts of agreeable and satisfactory surroundings, the gastric juice will differ materially from that secreted if one is eating under the stress of anxiety, fear, anger, etc. From this standpoint, the habit of having music at meals, and the jesters of olden time monarchs, have their physiological results. Modern psychotherapy can also be made of utility, in relieving a patient's mind of fear concerning his trouble, or anxiety regarding the proper selection of his food.

A moderate amount of fluid, especially water, has some influence in causing secretion of gastric juice, of a low digestive power it is true, but yet of some value.

Bitter substances taken before meals are apt to cause a desire for some succulent food, for the purpose of removing the taste from the mouth. Such food has an effect of this kind both by physical absorption of the bitter substance and by stimulating a secretion of the salivary glands which washes it away. This two fold effect thus causes a condition identical with appetite, and so, indirectly, stimulates secretion and digestion.

Foods somewhat tart and pungent have the effect of stimulating the nerve terminals, causing appetite and secretion.

Agents reducing gastric secretion.—A lack of appetite is the most powerful. If food is eaten without any desire for it, secretion and digestion are much less than if appetite is present.

It has also been shown that oil, taken before, during or after eating, materially lessens secretion of gastric juice. Whether this results from covering the mucous membrane, thus mechanically obstructing the ducts leading from the peptic glands, or reflexly by stimulating the inhibitory nerves of secretion, is uncertain, but it is supposed to be the latter. The fact that it has such effect, can be made of much service in treating cases of excessive secretion. Patients having such abnormality may begin meals with some oil, instead of bouillon as do those having decreased secretion.

Any agent which increases activity of the mucous glands lining the stomach, both reduces secretion of gastric juice, and by the alkalinity of the mucus secreted, very materially reduces the acidity and digestive power of what is secreted. Thus in experiments on dogs, solutions of mustard, pepper, nitrate of silver, etc., if used strong enough, will by their irritative properties on the mucous glands stop the flow of gastric juice entirely.

Alkalies, as sodium bicarbonate and magnesia have been accused in the past of increasing gastric secretion, but by physiological experiments on dogs, it has been shown that such is not the case. Instead they very materially decrease it. This fact is of extreme importance in treating excessive secretion, and its recognition has resulted in much benefit in such conditions.

The irritation of some nerve to such an extent as to cause pain, or some such painful affection as sciatica, will materially lessen gastric secretion. This it is well to remember in case a patient under observation develops such a condition. Possibly it may also be recalled to advantage in treating hyperchlorhydria.

GASTRIC ABSORPTION.

The absorptive power of the stomach is very limited, except for a few substances, and it is not often of much benefit to make examination in regard to this function. If it is desired to do so, the usual way is to give the patient a few grains of potassium iodide. A strip of filter paper, saturated with a starch solution and dried, is then moistened in the saliva every few minutes. As soon as the potassium iodide has been absorbed and carried to the salivary glands by the blood, it is secreted in sufficient amount to color the starch paper blue. This reaction normally occurs in from ten to fifteen minutes.

GASTRIC MOTILITY.

The motor function of the stomach, or, more correctly, the ability of the stomach to empty itself, is of considerable importance. This ability was formerly thought to be entirely dependent upon the integrity of the muscle fibres in the stomach wall. It has now been shown, as will be seen when studying the subject of motor insufficiency, that this inability is not always due to muscular weakness, but, when not due to organic stricture of the pylorus, is frequently a result of a spasmodic contraction of the pylorus, preventing an outflow of chyme from the stomach. This spasmodic condition is due to a duodenal reflex, acting automatically from the presence of too acid a chyme on the mucous membrane of the duodenum. However, this fact does not change the method for determining when the stomach empties itself.

For all practical purposes, simple lavage at stated times after a meal is all that is necessary. For instance, after a test breakfast, if the stomach is examined in an hour and found to be empty, evacuation is too hurried. On the other hand, if in two hours there is still part of the food present, evacuation is delayed. The same statements can be made in regard to the test dinner, performing lavage in three hours, and in six hours after eating. Another test is to give salol. This is not decomposed in acid solutions, therefore it remains unchanged until it has passed out of the stomach into the intestine. It is then split up unto phenol and salicyluric acid. The latter is immediately excreted by the kidneys, and may be detected by its giving a violet color on the addition of a neutral ferric chloride.

In determining the size of the stomach, palpation and percussion, both in the empty and distended condition may be sufficient. Distention may be induced by water, by pumping the stomach full of air through a stomach tube, or by giving the patient a teaspoonful of tartaric acid dissolved in half a glass of water, and by immediately following this with the same amount of bi-carbonate of sodium. This gives rise to rapid development of carbon dioxide gas in the stomach, so distending it that percussion may be satisfactorily employed. Transillumination of the stomach through the abdominal walls by means of a gastro-diaphane may also be employed. This consists of a small electric light on the end of a stomach tube, which is passed into the stomach, the other end, by means of fine wires being connected to a battery. The light thus being in the stomach is sufficient to give quite a clear idea as to its size and location, especially in those persons having thin abdominal walls. Another way is to give the subject a large dose of bismuth sub-nitrate suspended in water, and then to skiagraph the stomach region.

CHAPTER II.

DIETETICS.

As the chief function of the gastro-intestinal tract is the reception of food, and the accomplishment of the first changes in its progress into tissue and energy, it will be well at this time to consider somewhat the foods themselves, and to give some thought both to their composition, and to their uses in the body.

Broadly speaking, foods may be divided into five classes: —

1. Water.
2. Mineral matter.
3. Protein.
4. Fat.
5. Carbohydrates.

As about two-thirds of the weight of the body is composed of water, this is required in larger amounts than any of the other classes. The gastro-intestinal tract is not called upon to perform any chemical changes, or so-called digestion upon water. Absorption however is necessary, and this occurs chiefly after the pylorus is passed. Plain water is absorbed but to a limited extent in the stomach, but the addition of certain agents, especially alcohol will somewhat increase its absorption. The chief uses of water are to unite with other compounds and form tissue, to form a carrier by which other foods may be transported to the portion of the body where needed, and to carry excrementitious products out of the body through the eliminative organs. As a force producer it is probably of no value.

The mineral matter is found in compounds of sodium, potassium, magnesium and iron. These compounds also require no digestion, but are simply absorbed as found in various kinds of foods. They are used partly in the construction of tissues, especially the bones and teeth, and to some extent in all the soft parts. A very important function which they have is in connection with the chemical changes and activities occurring in the body. Five to six per cent. of the body weight consists of mineral matter.

Protein includes those foods containing nitrogenous compounds. They compose about 18% of the body weight. These compounds may be divided into three classes,—albuminoids, gelatinoids and extractives. The first of these may be either of animal or vegetable derivation. If the former they may be found in lean muscle fibre, white of egg and casein of milk. Examples of vegetable origin are gluten and cellulose found in cereals and vegetables. The gelatinoids are derived from the connective tissue of meats. The use of these two classes is to build tissue; either that required for growth as in the case of the young, or for the repair of old and broken down tissue. They are also used for fuel; that is, the carbon contained in them is oxidized in the body, thus generating heat and energy. Lastly, they are to some extent stored up in the body in the form of fat, as well as in the form of nitrogenous tissue.

The third class of nitrogenous compounds, the so-called extractives are considered as protein, because they contain nitrogen. They are found in meat and blood. Their chief and possibly only use are as stimulants and appetizers. They neither enter into the formation of tissue, nor do they generate heat and energy. Vegetable foods contain compounds of so-called amids, whose uses are similar to the extractives found in meat.

Fats are found both in animal foods, such as meats, cream and eggs, and also in such foods from the vegetable kingdom, as olives, cotton seed and some of the cereals. Fat gaining access to the body by means of such foods, may either be oxidized as fuel, or stored up as fat. Protein and the carbohydrates may also be changed into fat by the processes of metabolism, and stored as such in the body. The amount so stored differs widely, depending partly upon the amount of food eaten, and the amount of exercise taken; also partly upon individual idiosyncrasies, which are as yet not understood. In the average person the fat constitutes about 15% of the body weight. In conditions where for some reason sufficient food is not eaten to supply the body with heat and energy, this stored fat is the first and chief of the body tissues to be drawn upon to supply the deficiency.

Carbohydrates are found chiefly in vegetable foods, in the form of such compounds as sugars and starches. Of the animal foods in which they are found, milk is the principal one,—lactose or milk sugar constituting quite a prominent part of the solids found in this fluid. As tissue builders in the body, carbo-hydrates are practically unused, less than 1% of the body weight being composed of them. However, as said before, metabolism may change them into fat, and thus indirectly they become incorporated in the body structure. For the purpose of generating heat and energy they are of great utility.

As outlined in the preceding paragraphs, it may be seen that foods are eaten partly for structural purposes, and partly as heat and energy producers. The nitrogenous compounds, or protein are the tissue builders. Therefore the importance of eating them in sufficient quantity to keep the organs and structures supplied with repair material. Yet if eaten too freely there result certain by-products arising during the process of metabolism, which are deemed injurious to the organism, and have some causative influence in the production of certain diseases. Authorities differ as to what constitutes the proper amount for an individual, and of course much depends upon circumstances; such as the size of the person, the amount of exercise taken, the degree of temperature he lives in, and the amount of fats and carbohydrates eaten. For a healthy man, of average size, doing a moderate amount of work, and eating a proper amount of fat and carbohydrates, the average amount estimated by various authorities, is about 120 grammes per day. The only method of judging whether one is getting sufficient protein, is by determining whether his tissues are keeping well nourished. If it is decided that they are not, then the question arises as to whether an insufficient amount of albumen is not being taken, or whether the processes of digestion and assimilation are not taking care of what is ingested. If too much is eaten for a protracted time, it is usually evidenced by the symptoms of certain diseases caused thereby.

As nitrogen is an essential element in compounds used for tissue building, so carbon is necessary in those intended to keep the body warm, and secondarily, supply it with the energy to work. The fats and carbohydrates are especially adapted to such purposes; although as protein contains carbon as well as nitrogen, it also is used to some extent. Indeed, in case of necessity, or in carnivorous animals, it may be all that is essential. The amounts of these compounds needed are also variously estimated, but the proper consumption is probably about 90 grammes of **fat**, and 330 grammes of carbohydrates each twenty-four hours. To these amounts of albumen, fats and carbohydrates, about 745 grammes of oxygen from the air by respiration, about 2,818 grammes of water, and about 32 grammes of minerals are needed each day.

In computing the amounts needed to keep up heat and energy, a unit of measurement called the calorie is used. A calorie is the amount of heat required to raise the temperature of one kilogram of water, 1 degree Centigrade. Or, expressing it in terms used by mechanical engineers, one calorie is equal to about 1.54 foot tons. The number of calories needed each day by an individual, depends upon their size, the amount of exercise taken, the temperature of the atmosphere and other things. For a man of average size, exercising moderately and in a medium temperature, food yielding about 3,200 calories is needed each day. The number of calories which may be generated from a given quantity of the various foods, has been determined by means of an apparatus called the calorimeter. This consists of a copper walled chamber of sufficient size, containing furniture so that an individual may remain in it several days. During such time careful analyses are made of all food eaten, and of all the eliminations from the body by the breath and excreta. Also, a measurement is made of all energy given off in the form of heat and muscular activity. The difference between the food taken into the body, and what is eliminated, is called the balance of matter, and shows whether the body is gaining or losing material. The difference between the energy of the food taken, and that of the excreta and the energy given off is the

THE STOMACH

balance of energy, and equals the energy of the body material gained or lost.

By such tests the average nutritive values of some of the most commonly used foods, have been determined to be as shown in the following table:

AVERAGE COMPOSITION OF FOODS,
Farmer's Bulletin No. 142, U. S. Agricultural Department.

Food (as purchased)	Refuse	Water	Protein	Fat	Carbo-hydrates	Ash	Calories per lb.
	Per cent	Per cent	Per cent	Per cent	Per cent	Per cent	Cal-ories
Beef, fresh:							
Flank	10.2	54.0	17.0	19.0	-----	.7	1,105
Sirloin steak	12.8	54.0	16.5	16.1	-----	.9	975
Round steak	7.2	60.7	19.0	12.8	-----	1.0	890
Rump steak	20.7	45.0	13.8	20.2	-----	.7	1,090
Neck	27.6	45.9	14.5	11.9	-----	.7	1,165
Ribs	20.8	43.8	13.9	21.2	-----	.7	1,135
Fore quarter	18.7	49.1	14.5	17.5	-----	.7	995
Hind quarter	15.7	50.4	15.4	18.5	-----	.7	1,045
Beef, corned	8.4	49.2	14.3	23.8	-----	4.6	1,245
Beef, dried and salt	4.6	53.7	26.4	6.9	-----	8.9	790
Canned boiled beef	---	51.8	26.3	22.5	-----	1.3	1,410
Veal:							
Breast	21.3	52.0	15.4	11.0	-----,	.8	745
Leg cutlets	3.4	68.3	20.1	7.5	-----	1.0	695
Leg	14.2	60.1	15.5	7.9	-----	.9	625
Mutton:							
Fore quarter	21.2	41.6	12.3	24.5	-----	.7	1,235
Hind quarter	17.2	45.4	13.8	23.2	-----	.7	1,210
Pork:							
Fresh ham	10.7	48.0	13.5	25.9	-----	.8	1,320
Smoked ham	13.6	34.8	14.2	33.4	-----	4.2	1,635
Tenderloin	---	66.5	18.9	13.0	-----	1.0	895
Bacon	7.7	17.4	9.1	62.2	-----	4.1	2,715
Poultry:							
Chicken	41.6	43.7	12.8	1.4	-----	.7	305
Goose	17.6	38.5	13.4	29.8	-----	.7	1,475
Turkey	22.7	42.4	16.1	18.4	-----	.8	1,060
Beef Soup	---	92.9	4.4	.4	1.1	1.2	120
Tomato Soup	---	90.0	1.8	1.1	5.6	1.5	165
Cod Fish	29.9	58.5	11.1	.2	-----	.8	220
Mackarel, whole	44.7	40.4	10.2	4.2	-----	.7	370
Perch, dressed	35.1	50.7	12.8	.7	-----	.9	275
Canned salmon	---	63.5	21.8	12.1	-----	2.6	915
Oysters	---	88.3	6.0	1.3	3.3	1.1	225
Lobsters	61.7	30.7	5.9	.7	.2	.8	145
Eggs	11.2	65.5	13.1	9.3	-----	.9	635
Butter	---	11.0	1.0	85.0	-----	3.0	3,410
Whole milk	---	87.0	3.3	4.0	5.0	.7	310
Cheese, full cream	---	34.2	25.9	33.7	2.4	3.8	1,885
Condensed milk	---	26.9	8.8	8.3	54.1	1.9	1,430
Cream	---	74.0	2.5	18.5	4.5	.5	865

AVERAGE COMPOSITION OF FOODS. – Continued.

Food (as purchased)	Refuse	Water	Protein	Fat	Carbo-hydrates	Ash	Calories per lb.
Vegetable Foods:	Per cent	Per cent	Per cent	Per cent	Per cent	Per cent	Cal-ories
Entire wheat flour	---	11.4	13.8	1.9	71.9	1.0	1,650
Wheat flour, roller process	---	12.0	11.4	1.0	75.1	.5	1,635
Graham flour	---	11.3	13.3	2.2	71.4	1.8	1,645
Oat meal	---	7.7	16.7	7.3	66.2	2.1	1,620
Corn meal	---	12.5	9.2	1.9	75.4	1.0	1,635
Rice	---	12.3	8.0	.3	79.0	.4	1,620
Starch	---	---	---	---	90.0	---	1,675
White bread	---	35.3	9.2	1.3	53.1	1.1	1,200
Brown bread	---	43.6	5.4	1.8	47.1	2.1	1,040
Whole wheat bread	---	38.4	9.7	.9	49.7	1.3	1,130
Cake	---	19.9	6.3	9.0	63.3	1.5	1,630
Oyster crackers	---	4.8	11.3	10.5	70.5	2.9	1,910
Sugar, granulated	---	---	---	---	100.0	---	1,750
Beans, dried	---	12.6	22.5	1.8	59.6	3.5	1,520
Beets	20.0	70.0	1.3	.2	7.6	.9	160
Cabbage	15.0	77.7	1.4	.2	4.8	.9	115
Corn, green sweet	---	75.4	3.1	1.1	19.7	.7	440
Cucumbers	15.0	81.1	.7	.2	2.6	.8	65
Peas, green shelled	---	74.6	7.0	.5	16.9	1.0	440
Potatoes	20.0	62.6	1.8	.1	14.7	.8	295
Tomatoes	---	94.3	.9	.4	3.9	.5	100
Peas, canned	---	76.1	2.8	1.2	19.0	.9	430
Baked beans, canned	---	68.9	6.9	1.5	19.6	2.1	555
Apples	25.0	63.3	0.3	0.3	10.8	0.3	190
Bananas	35.0	49.9	.8	.4	14.3	.6	200
Oranges	27.0	63.4	.6	.1	8.5	.4	150
Watermelons	59.4	37.5	.2	.1	2.7	.1	50
Apples, dried	---	28.1	1.6	2.2	66.1	2.0	1,185
Figs, dried	---	18.8	4.3	.3	74.2	2.4	1,280
Almonds	45.0	2.7	11.5	30.2	9.5	1.1	1,515
Peanuts	24.5	6.9	19.5	29.1	18.5	1.5	1,775
Chocolate	---	5.9	12.9	48.7	30.3	2.2	6,625

It is necessary, therefore, to have a good general idea of the various kinds of foods, of their chemical composition, of the uses to which they are put in the body, and of their values as tissue builders or energy producers. It is necessary, moreover, to know their process of digestion, as regards the variety and the place of secretion of the gastro-intestinal ferment necessary for foods of different chemical compositions. It is not feasible, however, to form iron clad rules, or erect inviolable diet lists, built upon the chemical composition or caloric energy of foods, because personal idiosyncrasies, likes and dislikes, the effects of appetite upon the digestive secretions, and physiological problems as yet unsolved, enter into the question, and at times, make it necessary to select a diet which suits the individual case, instead of one which is in exact accord with chemistry. In other words a consideration of the diet for a patient must be equally considered from two standpoints:

1.—What does the patient need?

2.—What food can the individual patient utilize?

The practical application of dietetic principles will be taken up more in detail when considering the different diseases to which the gastro-intestinal tract and its accessory organs are subject.

CHAPTER III.

FUNCTIONAL DISEASES OF THE STOMACH.

Abnormal conditions of the stomach which are not associated with special anatomical lesions thereof, are considered as neuroses. They may be divided into three classes:—

1.—Sensory neuroses.

2.—Secretory neuroses.

3.—Motor neuroses.

GASTRALGIA.

Of the various forms of sensory neuroses, gastralgia is of most importance. This is a condition where pains occur in the gastric region, alternating with intervals free from pain. Such pains are not dependent upon any pathological condition of the stomach itself.

Etiology:—The varieties of gastralgia, are: —

1.—Gastralgia of stomachic origin.

2.—Central gastralgia.

3.—Neurotic gastralgia.

4.—Constitutional gastralgia.

5.—Reflex gastralgia.

Gastralgia of stomachic origin may follow the taking of foods that are indigestible, or that possess irritable qualities.

Central gastralgia occurs as a result of organic nervous disease. The one which most frequently causes it, is locomotor ataxia. In such a case the gastralgia is called a "gastric crisis."

Neurotic gastralgia refers to pains of the stomach which are present as a result of hysteria or neurasthenia. It is quite common in patients suffering from these affections.

Constitutional gastralgia is caused by some abnormal condition of the blood, due either to infection, intoxication or malnutrition. The infection most apt to cause gastralgia is malaria. The intoxications which may cause it are numerous,—such as lead, mercury, nicotin, uric acid and others. As examples of malnutrition gastralgia may be mentioned all forms of anæmia and chlorosis.

Reflex gastralgia may be caused by abnormal conditions of the uterus, ovaries and tubes, or in men by diseases of the genito-urinary organs. It may also be found as a result of other abnormal conditions, such as disease of the liver, kidneys, gall bladder and intestines.

Symptomatology:—The symptoms of gastralgia may come on suddenly, or be preceded by various prodromal signs, such as dizziness, nausea, salivation, headache and pressure in the region of the stomach. These indefinite symptoms, if present, are followed by intense pain. Most frequently it is of a cramping nature, possibly somewhat relieved by pressure; so that the patient is apt to be found in a doubled up position. Or the pain may be of a burning, cutting, or gnawing character. It is apt to radiate in different directions, as to the back, the sides, or the shoulders. The patient is anxious, extremities are often cold, face is pale, cold perspiration, small accelerated pulse which is possibly irregular. The attack may last but a few minutes, or for several hours. If of long duration, it leaves the patient prostrated, so that several days may be required to entirely recover from its effects.

Diagnosis:—In making the diagnosis it is important to decide:—

1.—Whether it is really pain of the stomach, or of some other organ?

2.—If it is certainly of the stomach, is it due to some organic lesion, or is it a neurosis? If it is a neurosis, of what variety is it as regards etiology?

Other affections which may resemble gastralgia, are:—

1.—Gall stone colic. In this the liver may be enlarged, and sensitive to pressure. The pain is extremely severe, and is apt to be felt in the back under the right shoulder. There may be a history of previous attacks, followed perhaps by clay colored stools, saffron colored urine, and possibly icterus; or, if the present attack has lasted long enough, these symptoms may develop.

2.—Nephritic colic may also simulate gastralgia, though usually in that condition the pain is lower down, more pronounced in the back and extends into the genitals and down the thighs. If there is doubt, examination must be made of the urine for traces of blood, crystals or other sediment known to give rise to calculi, as oxalates, phosphates or urates. The finding of these elements, however, can be considered only as suggestive of calculi, and not positive proof thereof.

3.—Rheumatism and myalgia of the abdominal muscles may resemble gastralgia; but these pains are aggravated by pressure and pinching, while gastralgia is apt to be relieved by such manipulation.

4.—The pains of intestinal colic may be in the upper part of the abdomen and resemble gastralgia, but as that condition is apt to be due to gaseous distention, there is found either diffuse or circumscribed tympanitis, and the pains are relieved upon the passing of flatus.

5.—Mistakes have been made in differentiating between acute appendicitis and gastralgia. Although the pains of appendicitis are first felt in the epigastric region, there is even at this time apt to be tenderness at McBurney's point, there is generally some fever and within a short time the pains are more marked lower down in the abdomen.

If it is determined that the pain is in the stomach, and that there is no organic lesion responsible for it, an attempt should be made to decide as to which of the etiological forms it belongs. This can generally be done by giving attention to the history, and the presence of other symptoms.

Treatment:—Fomentations, as hot as can be borne, and applied to the painful area, are frequently of much value. The galvanic current may be used, employing the hot application as an electrode, and attaching to it the positive pole. Drinks, as warm as can be taken will often be of benefit, employing either simple hot water, or adding ginger, peppermint, or bi-carbonate of soda to the water.

Colocynth 2x:—Is indicated in idiopathic gastralgia, with agonizing, griping pain, somewhat relieved by bending double. May come on after some strong emotion, at night or before stool. Is relieved during stool.

Dioscorea 2x:—Cutting pains, as though knives were thrust into the stomach, accompanied by a twisting sensation. May be relieved by bending the body double.

Cuprum 3x:—Cramping, cutting pains, may be caused by sudden turn or twisting of the body. Dyspnœa, pains extend to the extremities. Pain not relieved by heat.

· *Nux vomica* 3x:—Pain in morning, especially after too much food, alcohol, coffee, tobacco or sexual indulgence. May be accompanied by faintness. Pain may be clawing in character, relieved by hot drinks. Ineffectual urging to stool.

Kali carb. 3x:—Sharp, shooting, digging pains, extending into chest, or to the bladder and genital organs. Caused by cold drinks when overheated. Worse in damp weather. Pain comes during stool, and relieved when through. Worse from pressure, or from lying on the stomach.

Arsenicum alb. 3x:—Burning, boring, cramping pains, with anxiety and restlessness; aggravated or occurring with chill. Caused by cold drinks or ice cream. Especially useful when bordering on an inflammatory state, or occurring in anæmia.

Carbo veg. 3x:—Pains in evening after eating. Much bloating; caused by lactation or loss of any of the body fluids. Pains may be burning. Weakness, with tendency to collapse, with difficult breathing; coldness of body extending to the extremities. Pain temporarily relieved by belching.

Ignatia 3x:—Pains come on after fasting, from grief, or from fright. Relieved by eating. Pale face, and twitching of individual muscles.

Belladonna 3x:—Caused by sudden motion or jolting. Bending backward gives relief. Flushed face, dilated pupils. Pain so severe patient may go into convulsions.

Argentum nitricum 6x:—Most frequently useful for gastralgia due to locomotor ataxia. Gnawing, boring pain, radiating to the back and shoulders. Worse from eating; great flatulence; palpitation of the heart.

Pulsatilla 3x:—Pains before menses; worse in warm room or from rich foods. In girls with tendency to chlorosis.

Ferrum:—This remedy, given in material doses, will often be the most successful in cases due to anæmia or chlorosis. There is apt to be vomiting, possibly diarrhœa of undigested food. A pressing pain in the stomach extending through to the back. Much weakness, with dizziness, dyspnœa and tendency to faint.

OTHER SENSORY NEUROSES.

There are certain other abnormal sensations occurring in the stomach, not dependent upon organic changes, which although of not sufficient importance to be classified as individual diseases, yet may be mentioned as entities, sometimes of considerable interest.

Hyperæsthesia of the Stomach:—When there is an unpleasant sensation in the mucous membrane after eating ordinary foods. It may be a feeling of fulness or a burning. It is apt to occur in chlorotic girls and after alcoholic and sexual excesses.

Bulimia:—This is an excessive appetite, but one which can be satisfied. Occurs sometimes in hyperchlorhydria, ulcer of the stomach, tapeworm, hysteria, and tumors of the brain.

Polyphagia:—An appetite so excessive that it cannot be satisfied.

Akoria:—A condition where the sense of satisfaction does not occur. There may be no especial appetite, yet when the individual begins to eat there is no sense of having had enough. Cases have been reported, where seventy-five or eighty pounds of beef have been eaten in one day

Anorexia:—A condition where there is an entire absence of appetite.

CHAPTER IV.

SECRETORY NEUROSES.

When the secretory functions are not properly performed, there may result either a decreased or excessive amount of gastric juice, or of the ferments contained in such juice.

HYPOCHLORHYDRIA.

When occurring as a neurosis, hypochlorhydria is a disease in which, during digestion a gastric juice is secreted in which the hydrochloric acid is present in smaller amounts than normal. As a result of this, the pepsin and rennin enzymes are unable to perform their functions. It constitutes a form of nervous dyspepsia directly the opposite of hyperchlorhydria. As far as the gastric secretion is concerned, it is the same as is found in most forms of chronic gastritis, and in some cases of cancer of the stomach. The latter affections, however, have other symptoms, together with pathological lesions, which serve to differentiate them from hyprochlorhydria as a neurosis.

Etiology:—It is a secondary phenomenon occurring with neurasthenia, hysteria, tabes and various psychoses. In this respect, it resembles very closely its opposite condition of hyperchlorhydria, although it does not occur nearly so often.

Symptoms:—Occurring as it does only in connection with other diseases, it will be accompanied with the symptoms of such conditions. The symptoms depending upon the lessened secretion alone, may be slight or entirely absent, provided the motor function of the stomach is unimpaired. If that becomes weakened, so that food remains in the stomach longer than normal, then, owing to the absence of hydrochloric acid, fermentation takes place to an abnormal degree. This gives rise to flatulence and the formation of organic acids, which irritate the mucous membrane. The symptoms which the patient then experiences are variable and are simply those of imperfect digestion, and in many cases will so closely simulate those present in other affections, that a diagnosis can be made only by examining the stomach contents.

Diagnosis:—The disease with which it is most apt to be confounded, is chronic gastritis, but owing to the associated symptoms of a nervous character it can generally be distinguished; also, because like other symptoms of nervous affections of a functional nature, the digestive distress varies much in intensity. In chronic gastritis, however, the symptoms are generally of about equal severity at all times. By examining the stomach contents, the two troubles may be differentiated by the fact that in gastritis, besides there being a diminished secretion of the digestive ferments, mucus will always be present. In some cases of gastric neuroses, there will be a considerable variation in the amounts of the ferments found in the contents at different times. On some occasions they may be sub-normal, at other times excessive. Such a condition is called heterochylia.

Treatment:—To meet the nervous condition upon which the hypochlorhydria is dependent, it is usually best to nourish the patient well. As proteid foods are not acted upon to any extent in the stomach unless hydrochloric acid is present, they should be given in such a form that they may easily pass the pylorus, and come under the influence of the pancreatic juice. That is, they should be given in a finely comminuted condition. If pepsinogen is found to be present, as it frequently is, and even some-times if it is not present, much benefit may be obtained in improving nutrition, by giving the patient dilute hydro-chloric acid. It may be given in thirty drop doses of the dilute acid, in a glass full of water, slowly during the fifteen minutes following a meal. It was formerly thought that the only benefit derived from giving this acid in such conditions, was that the acid medium thus produced in the stomach made the otherwise inactive pepsinogen act upon proteid foods to some extent. Later experiments have shown that this is not the only advantage gained, but that the influence of the acid on the gastric and du-odenal mucous membranes, reflexly stimulates the pancre-atic secretion. It has also been found that, in hypochlor-hydria, the pancreatic secretion is deficient, as a result of an absence of the normal stimulus of the gastric secretion, and that the artificial acid thus given will then materially increase intestinal digestion. It is now thought that the greater part of the benefit obtained by such acid medica-tion is secured in this way instead of by improving gastric digestion itself. It has also been shown that other acids will to some extent have the same effect, but not to the degree that hydrochloric will.

The therapeutics applicable to the neurotic condition giving rise to abnormalities of secretion and the motor ac-tivities, are so similar, that they will all be considered to-gether, after having taken up the other affections.

CHAPTER V.

ACHYLIA GASTRICA.

Definition:—This is a condition in which the secretion of gastric juice is entirely suspended. It is comparatively rare.

Etiology:—It may occur as a neurosis, and for that reason is considered at this place, or it may be the result of entire destruction of the secreting cells in the stomach, resulting from gastritis, or other inflammatory changes.

Pathology:—If it occurs as a neurosis, there is no discoverable pathological lesion. If it is a result of inflammation, there is absence of the gastric glands, and therefore thinning or atrophy of the mucous lining of the stomach.

Symptomatology:—There being no secretion in the stomach, of course food is not acted upon except by the ptyalin of the saliva, until it passes the pylorus. It has been shown in experiments upon animals, that if there is no acid secreted in the stomach, or if it is immediately drained off through a fistula, the pancreas will not act to a normal extent. As a result of these abnormal conditions, mal-nutrition is apt to appear, which may progress to excessive prostration, emaciation and anæmia. In fact, destruction of the gastric glands, giving rise to achylia gastrica, was at one time thought to be the cause of so-called progressive pernicious anæmia. Although the two conditions are often found in a given case, later investigation has shown that this form of anæmia may exist, with the stomach still secreting.

Diagnosis:—Can be made positively only by examination of the stomach contents. In these there will be found not only an entire absence of hydrochloric acid, but also of the pepsinogens and rennin zymogens. The contents of the stomach will appear exactly as when eaten, except as regards the changes that resulted from the ptyalin and from fermentation.

Prognosis:—This varies. In some cases a careful diet, with plenty of acid drinks and other means of stimulating pancreatic secretion, will effect some relief, and a fair state of health may be maintained for some time, provided the motor power of the stomach is good, so that the food may be promptly passed on through the stomach. At other times perniciously anæmic conditions will arise, and treatment will not be of much avail.

Treatment:—In these cases it is not always possible to select a diet, chemically considered. In fact it is often best to be guided to a considerable extent, by the patient's likes and dislikes. In general an effort should be made to give as nutritious a diet as possible. It should be softened, or finely divided by running through a meat grinder, or by scraping. Fish, sweetbread and soft boiled eggs may be used. It is also well to take considerable liquid with meals or soon after, in an effort so to dilute the food that it can easily pass the pylorus. It may also be well to acidulate the liquids, so as to stimulate pancreatic secretion.

Therapeutics:—If the trouble is a result of a neurosis, the remedies mentioned at the end of this chapter will be most useful. If it is organic, and a result of gastritis, the remedies mentioned for gastritis will be the ones to use. If the symptoms of progressive pernicious anæmia develop, the methods recommended for that trouble will be needed.

CHAPTER VI.
HYPERCHLORHYDRIA.

Hyperchlorhydria, Hyperpepsia, Hyperacidity or Superacidity:—This is a condition where the stomach secretes a juice during the period of digestion, which contains more hydrochloric acid than is normal, or is compatible with a proper performance of digestion. The other enzymes may also be excessive, but as they do not produce symptoms they are not considered. There may or may not be an excessive amount of gastric juice. A modification called gastrosuccorrhœa is a condition where the gastric juice continues to be secreted even when there is no food in the stomach.

Etiology:—It is most frequent in adult males, although no age is exempt, and women quite frequently have it. It is more common in the well to do and educated classes, but is not confined to them by any means. Business and professional men with much on their minds are frequent sufferers, as also are those who use their minds a good deal in any pursuit, and perhaps do not take sufficient exercise. The influence of the mind in giving rise to abnormalities of secretion, both hyper and hypochlorhydria, is very marked. The habit of transacting business, or studying over business matters during the process of eating or soon afterwards, it has been shown, will markedly affect the quantity and quality of the gastric secretions. Possibly of still greater importance, is the habit of giving too much consideration to the various foods eaten at a meal from the standpoint of whether or not they will agree, and fearing that they will not. Food eaten under such circumstances, will usually cause distress, no matter how simple it may be. If the same individual, is situated in such happy surroundings that he forgets to be careful, and is free from his sense of fear, he may be able to eat food ordinarily considered much more difficult to digest, and have no trouble whatever from it. Hyperacidity is frequently but a symptom of some more comprehensive disease, especially neurasthenia and hysteria. It is often found in anæmia and chlorosis. It may be reflex from the eyes, genito-urinary system, diseased conditions of the bile tract, inflamed, adhered or sclerotic appendix, movable kidney, inflamed or fissured rectum, hæmorrhoids or pelvic diseases of women. In fact its presence is usually but a symptom, and is a part of an abnormal functioning of the nervous system, as shown also in other ways. Highly spiced foods, ice water and alcoholic drinks may assist in causing the trouble.

Pathology :—Being considered as a functional disease, no organic pathology is supposed to be present; but at times, perhaps as a result of the irritation by the over acid stomach contents, the mucous cells lining the stomach appear swollen, and may secrete a mucus. Some writers describe this condition as a separate entity, giving it the name of acid gastritis. The secreting cells of the gastric glands are at times larger than normal, possibly so much so as to give an hypertrophied appearance to the lining membrane.

Symptoms :—In typical cases, the pains are of a burning, gnawing character, and are at their worst from one to three hours after eating. There may also be a sense of faintness, waterbrash, or a feeling of a load or lump in the stomach. These various distressing sensations may usually be temporarily relieved by taking more food, a drink of water, or especially a dose of some alkali, as sodium bicarbonate or Vichy water. The appetite is frequently increased, and there may be much thirst. Flatulence is apt to be present. The mind is at times involved to some extent, there being a condition of despondency, melancholia and irritability. The tongue is free from coating, or nearly so, and is abnormally red.

Although the above are the most prominent symptoms of a typical case, yet, there are many in which the symptoms differ somewhat, so that it may be difficult to diagnose a case without an examination of the stomach contents. These, when removed in a case of ordinary hyperchlorhydria, will usually be larger in amount, and thinner than normal. This excessive amount was formerly thought to be due to too free a secretion of the watery elements, as well as of the ferments, and possibly, to an extent, and in some cases this is true. It is now thought, however, that such is not always the case, but rather, that the excessive acidity, by irritation of the pylorus, causes a spasmodic contraction, so that what is secreted remains in the stomach longer than normal, and so accumulates. This secretion, in the cases mentioned above as being sometimes called acid gastritis, may not appear very thin, but may contain sufficient mucus to be somewhat viscid and slimy. Under the microscope, it will be seen that the meat fibres are dissolved, but that undigested starch cells are numerous. The filtrate of the contents, when quantatively examined, will be found to have a total acidity of 70, 80 or even of 100; instead of being between 40 and 60 as they should be, and the degree of free hydrochloric acid will be above the normal which is 20 to 30. Perhaps this may reach 40, 50, or even 80. The albuminous elements of food will be found undergoing the normal process of digestion, but the starches will be almost unchanged.

Now let us compare the process of stomach digestion, as normally performed, with that occurring in a case of hyperchlorhydria. In the normal process, food taken into the mouth is mixed with saliva and the ptyalin immediately begins the digestion of the starches. This continues in the stomach until the hydrochloric acid reaches a degree of about 12. Twenty to thirty minutes should elapse before the free acid should reach this point. During this time, the starches have undergone a considerable amount of digestion. At this stage, however, this ceases, and a digestion of the proteids begins, as a result of the hydrochloric acid and pepsin which are now present. This proceeds until the food leaves the stomach for the intestine. Here it is made alkaline by mixture with the intestinal juices, and then the amylopsin takes up the digestion of the starches where the ptyalin left it, the fats are cared for, and the remainder of the proteids are digested by the trypsin.

In a case of hyperchlorhydria, when the food reaches the stomach, the hydrochloric acid is secreted more quickly and profusely than normal, and a degree of 12 is almost immediately reached. Hence, the ptyalin has scarcely any time to act on the starches. The digestion of proteids begins almost at once, and goes on rapidly. At the end of one to three hours the hydrochloric acid is so strong that the mucous membrane is unduly irritated thereby, causing the distress which is present at this time. When portions of chyme pass the pylorus they are so strongly impregnated with the hydrochloric acid that an irritation of the duodenal mucous membrane is caused, producing, as has been shown by experiment, the so-called duodenal reflex, and resulting in pyloric spasm with firm closure. Then no more chyme can leave the stomach until the intestinal and pancreatic juices and bile have produced a certain degree of alkalinity to exist again in the duodenum. As a result of these pyloric closures occurring more frequently than in cases presenting the normal degree of acidity, more time than normal is required for a meal of certain proportions to leave the stomach. Stagnation thus results, and the stomach is apt to become distended with food, gastric juice and gas. The latter results largely from fermentation of starches which have not been properly prepared, because the action of the ptyalin was of such short duration.

Diagnosis:—The diseases from which hyperchlorhydria will have to be differentiated, are gastritis, gastralgia, cancer, gastric ulcer, duodenal ulcer and duodenal adhesions.

1.—In gastritis there is more coating of the tongue, the appetite is lessened instead of being increased, the pain is less intense and comes on sooner after eating, there is a more offensive taste in the mouth, the symptoms are not modified by the patient's surroundings or mental attitude, and most important of all the hydrochloric acid is decreased or absent in the stomach contents, and there is mucus present.

2.—In gastralgia the pain occurs without regularity, and is neither temporarily relieved, nor followed later by aggravation upon eating. The hydrochloric acid may be normal.

3.—In cancer of the stomach or duodenum the duration of the disease is usually shorter, cachexia is more pronounced, the appetite is generally poor, pain is more steady, there seldom being much relief from it. Vomiting of small amounts of blood may occur, a tumor may be present, and the gastric contents as a rule show an entire absence of hydrochloric acid, and the presence of lactic acid; especially after much progress of the disease has taken place.

4.—In gastric ulcer the pains are more severe, and often radiate to the back, specially to the right of the twelfth dorsal vertebra. The pains come immediately after eating. Vomiting sometimes takes place, possibly of blood, although these symptoms are not necessary. There is practically always a very sensitive, circumscribed spot, which causes the patient to wince upon palpating the area. Gastric ulcer is almost always accompanied by an increase of hydrochloric acid, so that in many cases the symptoms of both conditions are present.

5.—Ulcer of the duodenum is often difficult to differentiate, because in this condition the occurrence of the pain is at the same period after eating, being caused by irritation of the chyme passing over the ulcer at this time. Accompanying duodenal ulcer there is practically always an excess of hydrochloric acid, but if ulcer is present, the pain is generally more severe and lancinating. There is a circumscribed spot usually a little to the right of the median line, and above the umbilicus, which is very sore to pressure. Patient examination of the fæces by the method given for that purpose will often reveal traces of blood. Alkalies will not give such entire relief to the distress felt as in hyperchlorhydria, but fifteen grains of orthoform will by acting as an analgesic to the abraded surface, often give almost entire temporary relief.

6.—Duodenal adhesions will also give rise to distress in the epigastrium, worse from one to three hours after eating. These are often the result of ulcers, and sometimes accompany them. If so neither the orthoform nor the alkali will give relief. If the ulcer has healed there will not be as marked tenderness on pressure. The distress present in adhesions is due to a dragging from peristalsis, which dragging is most pronounced when the chyme is leaving the stomach. The chief point in differentiating this condition from hyperchlorhydria is the failure to get temporary relief from the alkali.

Prognosis:—Relief from the trouble can generally be effected, but entirely remedying the condition and causing a return to the normal degree of secretion, is quite a difficult matter in most cases.

Treatment:—May be considered as psychic, dietetic, re-flex, chemical and therapeutic.

Psychic influence is of much importance in all forms of gastric neuroses, and especially in those of a secretory nature. These patients have usually suffered from their dyspepsia for a long time. They have tried diets of various kinds, until finally they have reached a point where all food is eaten with a sense of fear, and with the expectation that distress will follow. Food eaten under such circumstances, generally produces just what is expected from it. The first thing to do is by assurance, encouragement, argument, suggestion or whatever name may be given to psychotherapy, to impress upon the patient the necessity of eating sufficient food, of a mixed variety, in order to so improve nerve tone and general vitality that the stomach can do its work, and that any thing less than this is but aggravating the trouble; also that a meal of normal amount and variety will cause no more distress than the "tea and toast" or "chopped beef" or whatever they have been eating. If the matter is presented to them with the proper emphasis and encouragement to secure their confidence, and to alleviate their fears and anxieties, a test of eating a full meal of usual foods will prove to them the truth of the assertion. If they think that they cannot digest well, it can be shown them by testing for hydrochloric acid, and for the proteolytic power of their gastric juice, that instead of their stomachs being unable to digest food, they possess the ferments, and can digest even more than the usual amount, especially of the proteid foods. If these patients as a result of low diet in the past have gotten into a condition of malnutrition, anæmia or emaciation, the so-called rest cure is often of benefit. The rest, the isolation from friends who have been helping by their unwise counsels to aggravate their condition, and the opportunity which it offers the physician to educate the patient to a proper mode of living and eating, all tend to make this the ideal treatment in such cases.

The best way to give this treatment, is to put the patient to bed under the exclusive management of an intelligent nurse, who will follow the physician's instructions implicitly. The first week, a milk diet is usually best. If the patient thinks that milk does not agree, as he often does, this will generally be proven to him to be false, and the first step in securing his confidence is attained. After a few days of this, a return to a normal mixed diet will give the best results. If a temporizing method, of adding one article at a time is practiced, it only helps to fix false ideas in his mind, as to the comparative value, or digestibility of various foods. As examples of menus which may be given, the following may be suggested, although it is desired to insist emphatically, that in these various forms of indigestion due to neuroses, no iron clad diet lists are advisable. Be sure to order enough to nourish the patient well, but do not give too much attention to chemical or caloric values. Instead, eradicate from the patient's mind the necessity for giving such close attention to these details. As mentioned in the chapter on dietetics, the various classes of foods are to a considerable extent interchangeable as regards their uses in the body. As one of many samples for a breakfast, order a cereal well covered with cream. The fat of the cream, it has been shown by physiological experiment, inhibits the action of the gastric glands, and at the same time materially helps the nutrition. This may be followed with toast or dry bread, using butter freely, and also bacon, an egg or two, or a chop, and finishing with some fruit, and cocoa, chocolate or a glass of milk. In the middle of the forenoon give another glass of milk. Midday is the better time for patients taking the rest cure, to have their dinner, for if taken in the evening it may interfere with their night's sleep. For dinner, if the acidity is considerable, it is well to begin with a dose of olive oil or some plain oil salad, for the same reasons that cream was eaten at breakfast. Continue with some meat, as fish, beef or mutton, together with potatoes and other vegetables, as peas, green beans, celery, lettuce without vinegar, radishes, squash, cauliflower, stewed onions, in fact almost any of the ordinary vegetables, bread with plenty of butter, and tea, cocoa, or milk. For dessert, some plain pudding, stewed fruit, or ice cream may be eaten. In the middle of the afternoon give another glass of milk. For supper it is better to eat rather lightly of toast, or dried bread with stewed fruit, and a glass of milk. In the evening before going to sleep another glass of milk may be given.

Many of these patients will have been suffering from a degree of constipation that has caused them much worry, and will have been resorting to all kinds of laxatives and cathartics. Generally the free diet given above, together with assurances that no harm will result if their bowels do not move for a few days, will be all that is necessary to correct this condition. When the intestinal tract has really become sufficiently distended with waste material, peristalsis will be stimulated, and the trouble will really correct itself. However, there may be exceptional cases where a mild laxative is advisable, for a time at least.

During this rest treatment, we may employ some of the physical methods, as massage, hypdrotherapy and electricity, but apparently their influence is more suggestive than real. If used, one precaution should be taken, and that is so to use them as not to direct the patient's attention to any one particular part of the body, or any one organ. If this care be not taken, the mind of the sufferer is kept on the abnormality of such part, and, with neuroses, this is just what should not be done. If such methods are used, their use should be only in a general way, with the expressed statement that it is only to improve general nerve tone and vitality. At the same time the patient should be impressed with the fact that all the food given him is for the purpose of building up the general nutrition; that it is only by so doing that the distress caused by his weakened digestive system can be removed. Sleep should be induced in most cases simply by encouragement and suggestion, although in exceptional cases it may be well to get the patient started to sleeping by the use of some mild hypnotic, if he has been sleeping poorly.

In the class of cases mentioned, this line of treatment, rest, isolation, good feeding and education, carried out for six or eight weeks, will work wonders in improving a patient's health, relieving anæmia, malnutrition and neurasthenia, and the symptoms of hyperchlorhydria which are so frequent in these conditions. A return to activity should be made slowly, impressing upon him the necessity for keeping up his eating, and many other habits to which he has become accustomed during the course of the treatment.

Quite a large number of patients will be found, however, who are not anæmic, and who do not need the rest treatment. These should be examined carefully to discover if possible any trouble which is acting reflexly, or constitutionally by keeping them in the abnormal condition. If there is eye strain, gynæcological or genito-urinary troubles, evidences of bile tract or appendicular inflammations or adhesions, a movable kidney, rectal diseases, or any of the conditions mentioned in the etiology, they should be attended to, surgically or otherwise. The class of cases to which the rest treatment is appropriate, may of course also need surgical measures, but in such cases the best time for doing such work is often a matter requiring most careful consideration. It is a fact that the condition of neurasthenia is often aggravated by the shock resulting from an operation. Therefore it frequently is better to improve their general health by rest and feeding, before attempting any surgery. At other times, the existing lesions may be so prominent, and their influence so marked, that it is wiser to let the rest follow the operation. In any case after looking for, and attending to any reflex causes that may present, thought should be given to the possibility of the presence of any habits which may be producing a waste of nerve energy. One habit, which is apt to be undetected because of its nature, and which has a pronounced bearing, surprising in extent to one who has not been in the habit of carefully looking for it, pertains to sexual matters. In many neurasthenic and hysterical cases, associated with hyperchlorhydria, if thorough and judicious questioning is employed it can be discovered that sexual intercouse has either been indulged in too freely, or in some unnatural manner. This is a delicate matter upon which to get trustworthy information from a patient; especially a woman, but it can be done in most cases if properly approached. Many times it has seemed that a part at least of the benefit from a course of the rest treatment, has been due to the removal of a wife, for instance, from the excessive or abnormal embraces of a husband. In men also, such habits may either so prostrate, or else keep them in such an erethistic state, that the nervous force to the digestive functions is materially affected.

Attention should also be given to other habits, such as worrying, excessive mental work, etc. In cases not needing the rest cure, psychic treatment may also be of much benefit. They should be taught the advantages of a proper frame of mind during the process of eating and digestion; the wisdom of not selecting foods too carefully, with anxieties as to whether they will cause distress or not; the necessity of keeping the mind on other and pleasant thoughts while eating and afterwards, and that if any distress should be manifesting itself, they must try in every way possible to "forget it."

Possibly this method of treatment will meet with the disapproval of some, and even appear somewhat similar to that promulgated by the so-called Christian Scientists. In proper cases, however, if one will employ it correctly, and compare results with those attained under the older methods of carefully selecting each article of food for such patients, cautioning them to be careful about eating this and that, and finally leaving them only a few undesirable and non-nutritious articles which they are permitted to eat, one can not help but be impressed with the superlative value of this method. Of course, one must be sure of his case before instituting such treatment, and advising such liberal diet, and not make the mistake of employing this method when there really is some organic disease of the stomach, as gastritis, ulcer or cancer, but in every day practice, at least three cases of stomach trouble out of every five, are functional instead of organic, and the large majority of such functional cases are hyperchlorhydria.

In summarizing the psychic, hygienic, reflex and dietetic forms of treatment appropriate in this class of troubles, it may be said that, after correcting injurious mental impressions by education, instituting correct hygienic habits by advice, attending surgically or otherwise to any cause acting reflexly from a distance, the dietetic regimen in purely functional cases of hyperchlorhydria may be attended to by giving heed to the four following rules:

1.—Be sure the patient eats enough to keep up a good state of nutrition, without going to the other extreme of eating more than is needed.

2.—Give proper attention to the organs of elimination, so that auto-intoxication will not develop.

3.—Give a rather larger amount of fat than normal, both for its nutritive value, and for its inhibitory effects on secretion from the gastric glands.

4.—As ptyalin activity is limited in these cases, have all carbohydrates very thoroughly cooked, so they will not be as apt to undergo fermentation before reaching the duodenum and coming under the influence of the pancreatic juice. It is probably also well in many cases to somewhat reduce the amount of carbohydrates, partly because they do not digest well where there is so much acid, and also because the increased fats help to take their place.

The chemical treatment, if necessary to employ any, will consist in the giving of some alkali. It is only palliative in effect, and unless the excess of acid present gives rise to considerable distress it probably will be better not to give it; but if such distress does exist, the patient can be made to feel much better by giving an alkali, preferably from one to three hours after eating when the acid is at its highest point, and the discomfort is greatest. Plain bi-carbonate of soda, or equal parts of this and calcined magnesia, given usually in teaspoonful doses will often answer the purpose very well. Vichy water is also a good preparation to use for the same purpose. A prescription which is very satisfactory consists of the formula:

℞.

Magnesia usta,

Sodii carbon exsiccat. aa 1 part.

Sodii bi-carbon,

Elæosacch. menth. pip. aa 3 parts.

Sig.—Mix. Take a teaspoonful in a little water, two hours after eating. If constipation demands attention, 1 part pulv. rad. rhei. may be added.

Therapeutics:—As secretory and motor troubles of the stomach are so simliar in etiology and symptoms, and in fact so frequently exist together, it seems more desirable to wait until after considering the motor affections before taking up the important subject of therapeutics.

CHAPTER VII.

MOTOR NEUROSES OF THE STOMACH.

MOTOR INSUFFICIENCY.

Abnormalities of the motor function may present in any one of the four forms:—

1.—Increased peristalsis. This, if unaccompanied by pyloric obstruction, will result in a premature passage of food from the stomach into the intestine.

2.—Decreased peristalsis. This will result in stagnation of food in the stomach.

3.—A mixed, or combined increased and decreased motor activity.

4.—Reversed peristalsis. This sometimes occurs as a neurosis simply, and sometimes will develop in the earlier stages of pyloric obstruction. It is rare, and practically is not of much importance, unless it is considered in its transient form, as a part of the process of vomiting. Even here it has been found that the diaphragm and abdominal muscles are of more importance in expelling the food from the stomach upward, than is the reversed activity of the stomach itself.

Increased peristalsis, as an entity, is also quite rare, although cases occasionally present in which the food does not remain in the stomach a normal length of time. Instead of this being due to an increased peristalsis, however, it is probably more often due to a relaxation of the pylorus. The passage of food into the intestine thus not being guarded against to a normal degree, even the ordinary motor movements would evacuate the stomach in a period shorter than otherwise. Increased peristalsis associated with some other condition, usually pyloric obstruction, either spasmodic or organic, is a very common occurrence. When so complicated, instead of resulting in a premature removal of food from its cavity, the obstruction is generally such that, in reality, there is delay. The condition may be compared to cardiac hypertrophy, with increased force of the heart beat in an effort of nature to overcome an obstruction resulting from some diseased condition of an orifice. If a patient's abdominal walls are thin, peristalsis at such times may become so strong, that its movements may be seen by the eye, or felt by the hand. As said above, when obstruction is marked, the movement may become reversed. This is called anti-peristalsis, and when present seems to begin at the pyloric extremity and work toward the cardia. Usually this does not continue long, but soon develops into a condition where the muscle fibres become exhausted, and the second form of motor abnormality develops, viz., decreased peristalsis.

In the recent past, motor insufficiency of the stomach was thought to be of very frequent occurrence. Later experiments have shown, though, that as a primary condition it is much more rare than was supposed. However, it is quite apt to develop secondarily to other affections, especially pyloric obstruction. In fact many of the cases which in the past were thought to be insufficiency, or idiopathic dilatation, were in reality secondary to spasmodic contraction of the pyloric valve, due to the irritation from an over acid chyme.

Independent peristaltic inactivity is undoubtedly sometimes present. When so, it is usually due to a generally prostrated condition such as may exist in cases of profound anæmia, neurasthenia or a state of muscular weakness caused by some such disease as tuberculosis, cancer, nephritis, diabetes or organic heart disease. At such times its consideration would properly be with such disease, although, in anæmia and neurasthenia, attention may be demanded by such complication itself before proper nutrition can be taken and assimilated to overcome these conditions.

In the division where there is a combination of increased and decreased motor activities may be considered that class of cases in which, together with an undue contraction of the pyloric valve, possibly associated at first with increased peristalsis of the rest of the stomach wall, there finally develops a condition where, although the pylorus remains overactive, the rest of the stomach relaxes, possibly dilates, and its motor function becomes inert. This state of affairs is very common, and is practically always associated with hyperchlorhydria. It was Pawlow who showed that the mucous membrane of the duodenum possesses certain reflex centres which automatically close the pyloric valve when the amount of hydrochloric acid that can be properly neutralized by the alkaline intestinal juices has entered this division of the intestine. If the chyme entering the duodenum is over rich in acid, then only a smaller amount than normal can pass before the valve is closed, and it remains closed until the acid is neutralized when it will reopen and the process be repeated. It will thus be seen that in hyperchlorhydria the stomach contents are delayed in their passage to the intestine. Experiments on dogs made through a fistula leading to the duodenum, have shown that an injection not only of hydrochloric acid, but also of any other kind of acid will produce the same effect, to such an extent even that if the stomach contains nothing but plain water or a solution of bi-carbonate of soda, this can be kept there indefinitely, so long as an acid solution is kept in the duodenum to keep the pylorus tightly closed. On the other hand, injecting into the duodenum through such fistula, some alkali, as soda or magnesia, will cause an immediate opening of the pylorus, with rapid passage of the stomach contents into the intestine.

Knowledge of these facts has shown that in a large number of cases, motor insufficiency is but a sequel to hyperchlorhydria, and is not primarily a myasthenia or muscular weakness, although this too may develop later. It seems that at first, the same as in organic pyloric thickening, peristalsis is increased. If the patient's nutrition remains good, this "gastric hypertrophy" may partly at least, overcome the distress which would otherwise arise. But if the hyperchlorhydria becomes too intense, or if the patient's nutrition gets below par, then "compensation" fails and stagnation of the stomach contents arises.

In reviewing the various types of motor abnormalities, it is seen that all of them nearly always tend to ultimately result in allowing food to remain in the stomach longer than normal. Because of the terms motor insufficiency or gastric dilatation are often employed.

Symptoms:—When for any reason food remains in the stomach longer than normal, there is apt to be an unpleasant taste in the mouth, the breath may be offensive, and frequently the tongue becomes coated, especially at its base. A stomatitis or glossitis may develop. In most cases there is anorexia, though sometimes there is bulimia. Eructations of foul gases are common, sometimes accompanied with some of the acrid contents of the stomach. Unless cancer or ulcer co-exists, there is not apt to be very much pain, but more often a sensation of fullness, pressure and distention. Passage of food through the pylorus may be only retarded, yet in time it may all pass, or the stomach may be unable to completely empty itself, and so always may contain some food, even in the morning before eating. This condition is sometimes called ischochymia. Dilatation with ischochymia is nearly always accompanied with vomiting, which is of a characteristic variety. For one or two days the patient may suffer somewhat after each meal from an increasing feeling of fullness, then suddenly he will vomit abundantly, the ejected matter containing particles of food that were eaten at any time since the last vomiting attack. Its smell and taste are very offensive. After the vomiting there is a sense of relief until the next meal, when the same process is repeated.

Constipation is usually present and obstinate. As only part of the food eaten passes through the intestine, the stools are not only infrequent, but scanty. Where there is ischochymia, the urine is also deficient. The general health is injured to a considerable extent, because of malnutrition. The respiration and circulation may be interfered with, because of the dilated stomach crowding against the diaphragm. Where organic obstruction does not exist at the pylorus, ischochymia probably never exists.

Therefore, in such cases, there is not apt to be vomiting and the other symptoms are less severe. Those due to this condition alone, consist of a sense of fullness or distention lasting for a longer time after eating than is normal, unpleasant eructations, etc. However, as such cases are generally associated with excessive acidity, the symptoms of hyperchlorhydria are added to those of the food stagnation, and sometimes the spasmodic contraction of the pylorus mentioned as being caused by this extreme acidity gives rise to a sense of pain, somewhat resembling the pain of a gastralgia.

Chemical examination may reveal almost any secretory condition, although, as mentioned when considering the etiology, in the majority of cases there is an excessive amount of free hydrochloric acid. Many bacteria, sarcinæ, etc., are apt to be found under the microscope. The quantity of stomach contents is generally excessive, there being a greater amount of fluid than normal. There is also a tendency for the solid or food particles to settle to the bottom, leaving a large super-natant layer of thin fluid. On the top of this last layer, there is frequently a third layer, composed largely of the bacteria, sarcinæ and the lighter food particles. Owing to the abnormal fluidity, it has often been considered that there was a hyper-secretion, as well as a hyperacidity. Possibly there is some excess in the amount of gastric juice, in some cases at least; but evidently a decreased rate of passage to the intestine has more to do with the presence of the larger quantity. This, as explained before, is due to spasmodic contraction of the pylorus as a result of its irritation and a like irritation of the duodenal mucous membrane by the over acid gastric secretion.

Diagnosis:—Inspection will sometimes reveal the outlines of a dilated stomach. Percussion may also show that the stomach is larger than normal, or that its curvatures are not located as in a stomach of ordinary calibre. In employing percussion, it is often useful to distend the stomach, either by pumping air into it by means of an atomizer bulb attached to a stomach tube, or by giving the patient a powder of bicarbonate of soda, followed by one of tartaric acid. Lightly tapping the epigastric region with the finger tips will often give rise to a splashing sound, a so-called succussion sound. This has been considered to be heard only in stomachs in which the muscle tonus is impaired, and to be dependent upon the presence of both fluid and air in its lumen. In examining for this sound, as also in employing percussion, much care must be exercised in distinguishing between sounds arising from the stomach and those from the intestines, especially the transverse colon. The gastrodiaphane described in the chapter on examination of the stomach may be employed. In turning on the current, a zone of light as a result of transillumination of the abdominal walls, gives a pretty good idea as to the location and size of the stomach. The simplest and most satisfactory way of determining if the stomach is emptying itself in a normal period of time, however, is to employ lavage. If, two hours after an Ewald test breakfast, or six hours after a Leube test dinner, food can still be washed out of the stomach, it shows beyond doubt that there is delay. Methods should then be employed to determine if there is organic obstruction, or if it is functional insufficiency. These matters are considered elsewhere.

Treatment:—Motor inactivity due to anæmia, neurasthenia or other constitutional disease, is of course to be treated by remedying those affections. The more common form, really secondary to hyperchlorhydria, should in the main be treated identically with that condition.

Of considerable importance is attention to the diet. Chemically considered, this should in such cases be that recommended for hyperacidity. But, because of the weakened motor power, food should be as condensed as possible, so that its weight may not still further stretch the stomach walls. For the same reason, it should be taken in small amounts and more frequently than usual. Massage, electricity, and other mechanical means have been much employed; but, as it has been shown that in most cases the reason the food remains in the stomach too long is because of spasmodic contraction of the pylorus, there does not seem to be much benefit to be derived in thus trying to induce the stomach to contract more forcibly against the occluded point. Possibly such means employed in a general way, together with fresh air, exercises and hydrotherapy, may so benefit the general health that the hyperacid secretion will be reduced, and in this way they may indirectly be of assistance. The chief means, though, of overcoming the pyloric spasm, thus permitting the food to pass more freely, and so improving nutrition, is by the giving of alkalies. Those mentioned under the head of hyperchlorhydria, should be freely given at the time the chyme is passing into the duodenum, that is, from one to four hours after eating. Repeated doses at this time will give the best results.

The indicated homœopathic remedy should also be given faithfully, for its effect upon the general health, in this way seeking to make the organism perform its functions in a more normal manner. In the proving of our remedies, the gastric functions of secretion, motion, etc., were not investigated according to modern methods. So, in selecting the remedy, the only symptoms we have to guide us, are those of a subjective nature. As many of these symptoms are common to a variety of these digestive troubles, it will be more practical to group the therapeutics of both secretory and motor troubles at this place.

Nux Vomica 3x:—It is in functional digestive disorders that this remedy exerts its well known beneficent influences. Because of the fact that it will help so many such cases, however, it has undoubtedly been prescribed for many patients when some other remedy would have done better. The cases in which it is best suited are those resulting from alcoholic or dietetic excesses, or from the use of coffee, tobacco or strong drugs. Mental overwork with too sedentary a life. Tongue red, possibly sore, often coated yellow at the base. Bad taste in the mouth. Acid risings from the stomach; nausea and sour vomiting. Feels worse in the morning. Constipation, possibly alternating with diarrhœa. Stool difficult to expel, though there is a desire. Depression of spirits. Tension and fullness in the stomach. Great distress an hour or two after eating. Dull heavy feeling in the head.

Ignatia 3x:—After grief and worry. Tendency to melancholia, with desire to nurse it in secret. Hysteria and neurasthenia. Goneness in pit of stomach. Feeling of lump in throat, which cannot be swallowed. Eructations of bitter fluid. Aversion to tobacco smoke, warm food and milk.

Lycopodium 6x:—Excessive appetite which is easily satisfied. Excessive amounts of gas in the abdomen; acid eructations and heartburn. Desire to sleep after dinner. Tongue coated white. Constipation, with spasmodic contraction of anus. Urine scanty, with red sediment. Uric acid diathesis. Mind is despondent and apprehensive. Patient is weak and easily exhausted. Feels worse in latter part of afternoon.

Carbo Vegetabilis 6x:—The most innocent food disagrees and causes feeling of great distention with gas. Excessive acidity of gastric secretions. Gums bleed easily. Tongue coated white or brown. Extreme debility with cold extremities. Does not like meat, milk or fat foods. Griping pain, extending into chest. Gastric region sensitive to pressure, as result of being distended by gas. Sleepy during day, but cannot sleep at night, because of uneasiness and flatulence.

Phosphoric Acid 3x:—When due to sexual excesses. There is loss of appetite, with considerable thirst and desire for juicy fruits. Sour, acrid eructations. Feeling of weight in stomach after each meal. Red streak in middle of the tongue, which widens in front. Much weakness and exhaustion.

Kali Phos. 6x:—In functional digestive troubles connected with neurasthenia this is often a useful remedy. There is a nervous, "gone" sensation, soon after eating as though appetite was not satisfied. Empty, gnawing sensation, temporarily relieved by eating. Sour or bitter eructations. There is depression and weakness. Sensitive to noise. Easily frightened. Hysterical. Sleeps poorly because of "nervousness." Dreams a great deal, causing exhaustion.

Ferrum:—In anæmic patients, who are easily tired, and become breathless upon exertion. Poor appetite, sour risings, pale tongue and lips. Often long for acid foods, or chalk, lead pencils, etc. Frequent vomiting of undigested food. Constipated. This remedy often acts more promptly if given in material doses. For instance five grains of

Blaud's mass, or a few drops of Ferric Chloride in water after meals.

Calcarea Carb. 6x :—Milk disagrees, causing acid eructations. Unsuccessful efforts to eructate. Desire for hard boiled eggs. Thirsty at night, hungry in the morning. Much acidity; everything turns to acid; heartburn; offensive white stools. Acidity is the chief feature.

Anacardium 2x :—Faintness and bad feeling about the stomach, relieved by eating, but return in an hour or two. Tasteless or sour eructations. Desire for stool, but it passes away when an attempt is made. Weakness of memory and intellect.

Argentum nitricum 6x :—Stomach distended with gas, causing dyspnœa. Eructation is easy, and gives relief. Feeling of lump in throat, worse at night. Craves sweets, but they disagree. Flatulence after eating cold food. Especially useful in the indigestion of anæmic girls.

Sepia 3x :—Stone-like pressure in the stomach; sour putrid taste; desires acids. No inclination for stool for days at a time. Painful sensation of emptiness. Eructations worse after breakfast, and during menses. In women during the menopause.

China 3x :—Hungry, yet sensation of satiety. Flatulence, but eructations do not give relief. Much thirst; symptoms apt to be worse every other day. May have been exhausting discharges from some part of the body, or in nervous debility. Nausea with shuddering. May be distress about the liver.

Arsenicum album 3x :—Vital exhaustion and depression. Irritability of stomach with much thirst, and possibly nausea. Red tongue, with thin, silvery coating. Faintness; anæmia; emaciation.

Chamomilla 3x:—Painful pressure in stomach. Eructations aggravate and smell of food eaten. Thirst for acid drinks. In erethistic people who are hard to please; fretful and irritable. Pressure or burning at the stomach. Flatulence in upper abdomen.

Asafœtida 3x:—Much gas in the stomach, with foul, greasy eructations. Feeling of emptiness, with throbbing in the region of the stomach. Burning in stomach and œsophagus. Feeling in œsophagus as though peristalsis were reversed.

Pulsatilla 3x:—In chlorotic girls, or in people inclined to be stout, fair and of mild disposition. Distress from fat foods; yellow coated tongue, or may be white. Taste slimy or bitter. Feels as though stomach were overloaded. Throbbing or tingling in the stomach. Nausea with little vomiting. Heartburn.

Abies nigra 3x:—No appetite in morning, but great craving at noon and at night. Pain in stomach after eating, described by patient as feeling as though a hard boiled egg were in the stomach.

Alumina 6x:—When patient swallows food there is a sense of constriction which seems to interfere with the act. Starchy foods, especially potatoes disagree. Craving for indigestible substances as clay, chalk, and slate pencils. There is apt to be a paretic, and extremely dry condition of the rectum which produces marked constipation. Stools scanty and like sheep's dung. Patient apt to be of a neurotic temperament.

Sulphur 30x:—Hungry, with sense of hunger and faintness at 11 a. m. Feeling of emptiness an hour after eating. Eructation after dinner. There is much thirst, which is apt to be for something stronger than water. Waterbrash.

Colchicum 2x:—In patients of the uric acid or gouty diathesis, in whom there is much accumulation of gas, accompanied with a desire for defecation. Passage of mucus from the bowel. There is aversion to food, and the smell of it cooking causes nausea.

Iodine 6x:—As is quite frequently the case in hyperchlorhydria there is a ravenous appetite, but food seems to do no good. The patient remains emaciated. This remedy being recognized as acting prominently on glandular structures, should possibly be beneficial to the abnormally acting peptic glands. In some cases of complete absence of appetite in neurotic cases, this remedy in the 3x a few doses before a meal may promote a desire for food.

Natrum sulph. 6x:—In uric acid and bilious subjects. Thick and tenacious slime which must be hawked up. Bitter taste in mouth. Much thirst; stomach heavy and distended. Sour risings, heartburn and flatulence. Abdominal flatulence. Sallow skin and yellow eye balls. Headache with giddiness.

Phosphorus 6x:—Considerable appetite, which is apt to waken patient at night. Prefers cold food. Nervous exhaustion; patient easily tires; lack of ambition. One to five drops of a 1% solution of phosphorus in almond oil, taken after each meal is often beneficial in neurasthenic and generally debilitated patients, suffering from neurotic digestive troubles.

Robinia 2x:—A remedy for acidity. Eructations with sour fluid coming into mouth, which sets the teeth on edge.

Acid picricum 3x:—In neurasthenic people, who become tired on the least exertion. No desire to talk or do anything. Poor and capricious appetite. Thirst for cold water. Empty or sour eructations. Nausea and faintness.

worse on attempting to move about. Sensation of weight at epigastrium, with ineffectual desire to eructate.

Physostigma 1x:—Symptoms arising from irregular and spasmodic peristalsis of the gastro-intestinal tract. Resulting in colic, and sense of nervousness and trembling. No appetite, and especially dislikes cold drinks. Convulsive twitchings in all parts of the body.

CHAPTER VIII.
VOMITING.

The act of expelling the contents of the stomach through the œsophagus and mouth is done by means of an anti-peristaltic movement of the stomach walls, assisted by a contraction of the abdominal muscles pressing the stomach against the diaphragm, this latter having been made immovable by certain of the respiratory muscles.

Etiology:—In order that vomiting may occur, an afferent impulse must be sent to the vomiting centre, which is located in the medulla oblongata. Then an efferent or motor impulse is sent out, causing the necessary muscular movements. The afferent or exciting impulse may originate from almost any part of the body. Nearly all diseases and injuries of the brain may cause it. Certain affections of various organs, unpleasant odors or a swaying movement, as when in a boat may have such an effect. Irritation of the glosso-pharyngeal nerve, or gastric branches of the pneumogastric, or of the nerves supplying the liver, gall bladder, intestines, kidneys, genito-urinary organs, uterus or ovaries may cause it, as also may certain poisons, for example, uræmia acting through the blood. It frequently occurs in hysteria and neurasthenia, and is sometimes present in some of the infectious diseases, especially scarlet fever.

Diagnosis:—This has to do especially with the cause and character of the vomiting. In looking for the cause, an effort should be made to determine whether it is something originating in the stomach, or whether it is cerebral or reflex from some distant organ. If due to gastric irritation, there is generally nausea, and it is accompanied with pain and discomfort in the epigastric region, and with derangements of digestion. In cerebral vomiting, nausea is not apt to be so marked, in fact is sometimes absent, yet the stomach is unable to retain its contents. Instead, there may be vertigo, headache, and disturbances of vision, sensation and motion. There may be coma or convulsions. If it is due to reflex causes acting from some distant organ, or to irritation of some of the peripheral nerves, there are apt to be other sensations at the seat of the lesion which will assist in directing attention to the source from which the trouble originates.

As to the character of the vomited matter, if it occurs soon after eating, the food may appear nearly unchanged. If a longer period has elapsed it may be nearly digested, may present evidences of fermentation, or be mixed with mucus, indicating gastritis with pus or blood, indicating ulcer or cancer, with fæcal matter, indicating intestinal obstruction, or with poisonous substances.

Treatment:—The first thing to do is to try to discover the cause, and if possible remove it. If there are organic lesions of the stomach, they should be treated according to methods mentioned under such diseases. For the symptom of vomiting itself, rest should be enjoined; hot applications or sinapisms may sometimes be useful.

When vomiting is secondary to conditions of the central nervous system, the most frequently useful remedies will be,—

Helleborus niger 3x:—In vomiting from meningitis, after stage of effusion has commenced. Also in cases of hydrocephalus with vomiting. Patient being in state of dullness or stupefaction. Vomited matter apt to be greenish or black. Thirst for very cold water.

Aconite 3x:—Vomiting from cerebral excitement and congestion. Much erethism and anxiety. Bitter bilious vomiting, with cold sweat. Chilly. Apt to be useful in vomiting of scarlet fever.

Belladonna 3x:—Also useful in vomiting of cerebral origin, as of scarlet fever. Throbbing headache, dilated pupils, may be delirium. Vomiting may be but scanty, but there is much retching, accompanied with vertigo.

Arnica 3x:—After mechanical injuries, as blows or falls upon the head. Much gas in stomach, foul breath and stubborn vomiting, with throbbing headache and drowsiness.

Iris versicolor 2x:—Useful in vomiting of so-called sick headache. Vomited matter bitter or sour. Great burning distress in epigastrium.

When the vomiting is caused by inflammation, or irritants acting on the stomach itself, either within its cavity, or circulating in the blood and acting on the nerve filaments in its walls, another class of remedies will be useful.

Arsenicum album 3x:—Nausea and vomiting, with sensation of great weakness, distress and anxiety. After cold foods or drinks. Stomach feels full and distended. Griping pains in the stomach. The vomiting requires great effort, is scanty, and is followed by great prostration. It comes in irregular, spasmodic attacks. Vomited matter may be thin, or consist of glairy mucus. Useful in the vomiting of drunkards.

Ipecac 2x:—Distressing and intense vomiting of large quantities of water or stringy mucus. Preceded by profuse flow of saliva. Clean tongue; relaxed feeling in stomach. Vomiting is frequent, persistent and accompanied with great nausea.

Antimonium crudum 3x:—Vomiting due to overloading of stomach. Symptoms quite similar to Ipecac, except the tongue has a thick, milky white coating.

Nux vomica 3x:—Feels desire to vomit, but cannot. Would feel better if could vomit. May expel small quantities of sour, bitter matter. More apt to have the condition in the morning.

Pulsatilla 3x:—Nausea and vomiting from fatty foods, or from smell of cooking food. Coated tongue, white or yellow. Foul eructations. Pulsatilla temperament.

Phosphorus 6x:—Characteristic vomiting is of fluids as soon as they become warm in the stomach. Vomited matter may be only watery in these cases. But there are also other forms where a coffee ground matter is expelled.

Ignatia 3x:—Is apt to be useful in the vomiting of hysterical subjects. There is empty retching, only a little bitter fluid being expelled. Simple food may be vomited, while others that are ordinarily difficult of digestion will be retained, and possibly give relief to the nausea.

Veratrum album 3x:—Vomited matter comes forcibly, as though from a pump. Apt to be accompanied by a profuse and prostrating diarrhœa.

The vomiting of seasickness is most apt to be benefitted by,—

Cocculus indicus 2x:—Extreme nausea and vomiting. Vertigo. Worse from eating, drinking or in the open air. Vomited matter is acid.

Apomorphia 3x:—May also be useful in seasickness, especially if there is not much nausea, but there is profuse vomiting of thin water.

For the vomiting produced reflexly by conditions acting from distant organs, the remedies suited to the existing lesions of those organs will usually be of most service. However, ordinary stomach remedies will often be useful in relieving this symptom, even at such times; such remedies, for instance, as Arsenicum, Ipecac, Nux vomica, or Apomorphia.

In vomiting due to poisons, or severe irritants in the stomach, and temporarily at least in intestinal obstruction, lavage may be of much use. Pellets of ice, champagne, beer, 20% solution of cocaine, have all been used, sometimes with success. Occasionally only by obtunding the nerve centres by morphia, may relief from vomiting be secured. Of course this is only temporary, and as its effects are wearing away, the vomiting may return with increased force, yet in desperate cases temporary relief, even at this risk may be demanded.

CHAPTER IX.

HÆMATEMESIS.

Hæmorrhage from the stomach, or vomiting of blood, though but a symptom of some other disease, is of sufficient importance to demand special attention. Its most frequent cause is either ulcer or cancer of the stomach; but it may occur as a result of traumatism, from certain blood conditions, as a vicarious menstruation, or where there is great passive congestion of the mucous lining caused by obstruction to the portal or cardiac circulation.

Diagnosis:—This consists in determining whether blood really comes from the stomach, or whether it comes from some other source. A differentiation between blood from the stomach and from the lungs is most frequently demanded. Physical examination of the patient will usually determine which of these organs is the seat of the lesion. The quality of blood also differs. When from the lungs it is ærated and frothy, bright red, non-coagulated, and alkaline in reaction. When from the stomach these conditions do not exist. It is possible however for blood to first come from the lungs, be swallowed, and then arise from the stomach with these distinguishing marks destroyed as a result of the action of the gastric juice. The blood may also come from some portion of the intestine, mouth, throat or œsophagus. If so, it may be impossible to determine its source, unless some lesion of these various places can be found by physical examination.

Prognosis:—It but very seldom results in death, although it is quite an alarming symptom.

Treatment:—The most important measure is rest. General rest by quiet repose in bed, and local rest by refraining from food. Rectal feeding alone should be employed for a few days, and this should be followed by the most bland liquid, or semi-liquid food. An ice bag over the stomach may be of use, also the swallowing of small pieces of ice.

Ipecac 3x:—This will often be useful. The bleeding comes suddenly, and is accompanied by severe nausea, coldness and pallor of the face. Pulse weak, oppressed breathing, great thirst, blood usually bright red, but may be dark.

Secale cornutum 3x:—Passive hæmorrhage, blood is thin and does not coagulate easily. Great prostration, no pain; face, lips and tongue deadly pale. Cold sweat, quick, thread-like pulse, patient lies quiet and is not excited.

Millefolium 2x:—Especially if the result of traumatism. Bright red blood.

Hæmamelis 1x:—Fullness and pain before the hæmorrhage. Gurgling in the abdomen. Resulting from suppressed menses. There is vomiting of thin, rather dark blood.

Aconite 3x:—Vomiting of bright red blood, great anxiety with pain in stomach, or a sensation of coldness. The extremities are cold and there is a small, quick pulse.

Phosphorus 6x:—Especially useful in cases of hæmophilia. Bright red blood; drowsiness; pallor of mucous surfaces; empty gone feeling in the stomach. Urine dark, skin warm and moist. The coffee ground vomit often found in cancer of the stomach, is a prominent indication for phosphorus, or if this kind of vomit arises in ulcer, phosphorus will be of benefit.

Carbo vegetabilis 6x:—Body cold, Hippocratic countenance. Blood black and thick. Condition of patient very low.

Erigeron 3x:—A bright red vomit, made decidedly worse by every movement of the patient.

A solution of suprarenal extract or adrenalin may be of benefit, either given internally, used as lavage, or introduced directly into the blood stream hypodermically, or associated with a normal saline solution. If, however, the physiological action of any drug is demanded, the best results will be obtained by giving ten to twenty drops of ergotole, hypodermically.

CHAPTER X.
ORGANIC DISEASES OF THE STOMACH.
ACUTE GASTRITIS.

Definition:—An acute inflammation of the walls of the stomach, especially of the mucous coat.

Etiology:—The cause which most usually produces this disease, is some error of diet. This may consist in an excessive quantity of food eaten at one time, or in eating food the quality of which is not suitable to the individual. Excessive amounts may cause the condition not only by mechanical distention, but also because the stomach is not able to expel the contents until fermentation has occurred, with its resulting organic acids and gases, which act as chemical irritants. Foods which are eaten too hurriedly, without suffcient mastication, may cause trouble on account of the mechanical injuries done by coarse particles. Some foods are naturally of an irritating nature, and may produce acute gastritis by their mere presence. As examples may be mentioned alcohol, various condiments, and decomposed foods. Articles the temperature of which is either too high or too low may also irritate. Some people are peculiarly susceptible to certain kinds of foods; for instance strawberries, will in some people set up an attack of gastritis; in others, oysters will have the same effect. Besides the above causes, acute gastritis is a frequent accompaniment of certain of the acute, infectious fevers, especially scarlet fever.

Pathology:—There are two reasons why it is difficult to carry out a very thorough study of the changes which occur in this affection. One is that, uncomplicated, this affection very seldom results in death, therefore post-mortems are rare. The other is, that in cases that do die, auto-digestion of the cells lining the stomach begins as soon as life departs, so that at autopsy it is impossible to distinguish between the changes that were produced before death, and those which took place afterwards. The following from Woodhead's pathology is probably as good as can be given. "Distention of the blood vessels, often accompanied by small hæmorrhages, extravasation of leucocytes, and swelling and proliferation of the endothelial cells of the lymphatics, are the most noticeable points; epithelial changes as a rule being indistinguishable for the reasons above given, but when they can be made out, the epithelial cells contain large globules of mucin, are desquamating or undergoing disintegration changes, while the epithelial cells of the peptic glands are usually granular, and often detached.''

Symptomatology:—The first symptom to make its appearance, is usually a sensation of fullness or distention. There is much eructation, which at first gives relief, but later fails to do so. If the attack is a mild one, these symptoms may persist for a few days and then disappear. If the attack is more severe, nausea, followed by vomiting, may occur, accompanied by some pain in the epigastric region, anorexia, much thirst, and either constipation or diarrhœa. There may be headache and slight fever. There is considerable prostration, with possibly dizziness and much sweating. Herpes labialis is a frequent occurrence. When vomiting takes place, it consists of mucus, decomposing food, possibly bile, and in very severe cases, blood. On physical examination the stomach is found to be bloated and sensitive. The tongue is thickly coated. Temperature may be 102 or 103, or it may be normal. Urine is decreased in amount and of high color. Chemical examination of vomited matter shows entire absence of hydrochloric acid, and possibly the presence of organic acids, which are the result of fermentation.

Diagnosis:—In attacks that do not have fever, the diagnosis is usually easy, and consists in finding the cause, and the consideration of the above symptoms. The attacks which are accompanied with fever may be mistaken for some infectious fever, especially scarlet or typhoid. It may be distinguished from scarlet fever by absence of sore throat, appearance of tongue and absence of rash. In some cases, to differentiate between acute gastritis and typhoid is difficult and may be impossible for the first few days. The principal factors in deciding between them in the early stages are the temperature and the condition of the spleen. In acute gastritis the temperature rises rapidly, remains at about the same point for a time and then suddenly drops. In typhoid the temperature rises gradually, declining a little each morning and rising a little higher each evening. In typhoid there is usually enlargement of the spleen, which can be detected by percussion. After a few days it is easy to differentiate between these diseases, for then in typhoid there are the right iliac tenderness, the rose spots and the Widal reaction.

Prognosis:—The outcome is usually favorable, except in cases where it attacks children and aged people.

Treatment:—The treatment resolves itself into prophylactic, dietetic and therapeutic. The prophylaxis of course consists in avoiding the errors of eating mentioned in the etiology. In the dietetic treatment the best method is to avoid all foods for at least 24 hours, or possibly longer if the case is a severe one. At the same time it may be well to empty, as fast as possible, the gastro-intestinal tract, by such methods as lavage, and some mild laxative or an enema. To quench thirst small particles of ice may be swallowed during this time. After such period of rest it is best to begin with small amounts of liquid food, such as strained barley or rice water. If this is well borne, after a few hours beef bouillon, rice soup or oat meal gruel may be taken. As the appetite begins to return, soft boiled eggs, toast and other light semi-solid foods are permissible.

A diet of this kind protracted over a week, will generally bring about recovery except in very severe cases, when it should be continued for a longer time. If excessive prostration occurs, small amounts of brandy or champagne may be used.

Arsenicum album 3x:—Much nausea and vomiting; burning pains in the stomach and abdomen, with pale, anxious countenance, and cold sweaty skin, or may be dry and hot. Tongue dry and red, thirst for small quantities of water; great prostration; apt to be diarrhœa. Especially useful if caused by cold drinks.

Bryonia 3x:—Useful in hot weather, especially when caused by cold drinks. Sticking pains in stomach, worse on motion; dizziness when rising to feet. Tongue coated white, much thirst for large quantities of water. Constipation, stools being dry and hard.

Nux vomica 3x:—Caused by overeating, by alcoholic drinks, by emotional influences. Sour bitter taste in the mouth. Tongue coated white or yellow, especially at the base. Dull heavy feeling in the stomach; dizziness, frontal headache, irritable temper, worse in morning. Constipated, or constipation alternating with diarrhœa.

Ipecac 3x:—Much nausea and vomiting; bloating of abdomen and stomach. Tongue usually clean, but there may be some white coating. Apt to have been caused by sour drinks or foods, or by unripe fruit.

Antimonium crudum 3x:—There is also much nausea and vomiting, but there is a milky, moist white coating on the tongue. Much thirst, especially at night. Belching, with taste of food the same as when eaten. No fever.

Pulsatilla 3x:—Apt to have been caused by eating fatty foods, or pastry. No appetite, smell of food nauseates. No thirst, tongue coated yellow or white; edges feel sore; bitter taste in the mouth. Chilliness, stitching pain in the stomach, worse from pressure, motion or inspiration.

Other remedies that may be useful are,—Aconite, Belladonna, Gelsemium, or Baptisia in cases attended with fever. In other cases,—Podophyllum, Hydrastis, Chelidonium, Veratrum album, Chamomilla, Sanguinaria and Mercury.

CHAPTER XI.

PHLEGMONOUS GASTRITIS.

Definition:—An acute inflammation of the sub-mucous and muscular tissues of the stomach. It is a very rare condition.

Etiology:—There are two forms of this condition, viz: Idiopathic and Metastatic. The exact causes of the idiopathic form are not well understood, but it is probably the result of microbic infection. Traumatism, alcoholic excesses and dietetic errors seem to predispose to its occurrence. The metastatic form arises secondarily to pyæmia, puerperal fever, and the exanthematous fevers.

Pathology:—There may be a single abscess in the stomach wall, but more often there are several at the same time. Perforation may occur, either into the stomach or into the peritoneal cavity.

Symptomatology:—The symptoms are very acute, and consist of intense pain and severe burning in the stomach, with much soreness on pressure. Thirst, dry tongue and complete anorexia are present. There is high fever, (103° to 105°). Pulse small and irregular. There is usually nausea and vomiting. Bowels may be constipated, but usually there is diarrhœa. At last the mind becomes affected, and there is coma or delirium.

Diagnosis:—This is very difficult as the symptoms so closely resemble peritonitis. If in addition to the above symptoms we can determine one or more circumscribed spots in the stomach, which give increased resistance on pressure, we may think of phlegmonous gastritis.

Prognosis:—Very unfavorable, as most cases die in from three to five days.

Treatment:—The disease is so rare, and success in its treatment is so seldom attained, that no very definite line of treatment has been devised. But it would probably consist in rest, cold applications, and the use of Aconite, Belladonna, Bryonia, Mercury and Hepar sulphur. If diagnosed in time, operation may be considered, with the idea of incising the abscess and draining it.

CHAPTER XII.

TOXIC GASTRITIS.

This is an inflammation of the stomach that follows the ingestion of some irritant or corrosive poison. The principal agents thus acting are the mineral acids, caustic alkalies, oxalic acid, carbolic acid, corrosive sublimate, arsenic, phosphorus, and a few others.

Pathology:—Depends upon the variety, strength and amount of the poison swallowed. The first changes are the same as those in acute gastritis from other causes, or they may be more severe if the poison is sufficiently corrosive. The entire mucous membrane may be destroyed, or even the entire wall of the stomach may be perforated.

Symptomatology:—The symptoms will be more or less severe, depending on the character of the poison. If severe they consist in nausea, vomiting, thirst and pain. The vomited matter may contain blood. If the patient survives these symptoms, they may be followed by icterus, peri-

tonitis and hæmaturia. Later there may be atrophy of the
gastric glands, with absence of secretion. Occasionally
strictures occur, either in the œsophagus, in the stomach itself thus causing the so-called hour glass stomach, or at
the pylorus. Such stricture is the result of cicatricial contraction. Its period of development depends somewhat
upon the variety of poison taken.

Treatment:—There are three things to do in treating
these cases, viz.:

1.—Remove as much of the poison as possible.

2.—Antidote that portion which cannot be removed.

3.—Treat the symptoms resulting from the poison, with
the indicated remedy and such other means as may be
needed.

To meet the first of these indications, either the stomach
tube or a good, quick emetic may be used. The tube should
not be used if the poison was of an excessively corrosive
nature, as it might cause perforation of the stomach walls.
As an emetic, apomorphia 1/10 grain will usually act more
quickly than any thing else. Before vomiting occurs it is
well to give an antidote, or else dilute the poison with oil,
water or white of egg, so that in coming up it will not
cause so much damage to the œsophagus and pharynx. The
antidote should consist of some alkali, in case the poison
was an acid, and of an acid if the poison was a caustic
alkali. Demulcent drinks, as oil, milk or white of egg
should also be given after vomiting has taken place. Later
treatment does not differ materially from that applied to
other varieties of severe acute gastritis.

Mycotic, diphtheritic and other forms of gastritis, due
to bacterial infection of the mucous membrane of the stomach have been reported. However they are so rare, and
their diagnostic signs are so obscure, that merely mention

of their possibility will here be made. Their treatment would be symptomatic, by the indicated remedy, and if their specific nature could be determined, some antiseptic might be used as lavage.

CHAPTER XIII.

CHRONIC GASTRITIS.

Definition:—A chronic inflammation of the mucous lining of the stomach.

Etiology:—It may occur as a sequel to acute gastritis, or be a primary disease. A frequent cause is too rapid eating. Food is swallowed which has not been properly masticated and insalivated, and as a result the gastric mucous membrane is mechanically injured by the hard particles. Overloading the stomach may act as a cause not only by distending the stomach, thus interfering with the circulation, but also by the resulting formation of gases and organic acids which act as chemical irritants. Numerous articles of food and drink may produce chronic gastritis, as for example ice water, tea and coffee that are too strong, alcoholic liquors, tobacco and strong condiments. Carious teeth may act as a causative agent, not only because they interfere with proper mastication, but also because the food may become impregnated with products of putrefaction which have become lodged in such teeth. Chronic gastritis may result secondarily to other diseases, such as anæmia, chlorosis, scrofula, typhoid fever, diabetes, chronic diseases of the liver, kidneys, heart and lungs.

Pathology:—The region of the pylorus is most frequently affected, though the inflammation may extend over the whole surface, and may penetrate to the sub-mucous and muscular coats. The glands become enlarged, and the cells lining them granular; or they may undergo fatty degeneration. Great numbers of small cells develop, obstructing the mouths of the glands and causing retention of their secretions. In the earlier stages, the color is redder than normal, but later as a result of pigment metamorphosis in the blood corpuscles that have escaped from the vessels, the color becomes bluish or brownish. After a long time the glandular elements may become entirely destroyed.

Symptomatology :—In many cases the first symptoms are so slight as to be hardly noticeable. When they do attract attention, they are as follows:

Anorexia.—The patient may feel that the stomach is empty, but there is no craving for food, or if some appetite does exist, a few swallows of food satisfy it, and make the subject feel as though the stomach were distended. If there is a craving for anything, it is usually for some highly spiced food.

Taste.—In nearly all cases there is some abnormal taste. It may be described as metallic, bitter, sour or pasty. In some cases this is due to an associated catarrh of the mouth or throat.

Nausea.—Frequently this is present. It may be slight, or severe enough to cause vomiting. It is generally worse after eating.

Eructation.—This is nearly always present. May be only of gas, or some of the contents of the stomach may be brought up; a condition called pyrosis.

Pain.—This is not ordinarily present to any extent, but there is often a sensitiveness or tenderness perceptible upon pressure, which causes some distress after eating, although this distress is more a feeling of fulness or distention than of real pain.

Defecation.—In the majority of cases there is constipation, unless the condition is associated with enteritis, in which case there may be diarrhœa, or the two conditions may alternate.

Urine.—This is apt to be scanty, and contain a precipitate upon standing. Such precipitate usually consists of urates or phosphates.

General Symptoms.—The patient feels below par, both physically and mentally. Becomes tired easily, not having a normal amount of ambition. Sometimes there is more or less headache; or at least a dull heavy feeling, worse in the morning. There are apt to be cold extremities, and the patient chills easily.

Objective Symptoms.—The tongue is generally covered, either by a grayish white, or yellow coating, though sometimes a clean, red, irritable looking tongue is seen. On palpation, the gastric region is often found to be bloated and somewhat sensitive to pressure. If there is any liquid in the stomach, percussion is apt to cause a splashing sound.

Gastric Contents.—Mucus is usually present in excessive amounts. Hydrochloric acid is either absent, or present in diminished amount, except in the class of cases mentioned under the subject of hyperchlorhydria, in which the excessive acid seems to irritate the mucous glands to such an extent that secretion of mucus is stimulated. In such cases there will be an excess of mucus and also an abnormal degree of hydrochloric acid. Some authors classify this condition under a separate heading, called acid gastritis. However, in the vast majority of cases if mucus is present, its alkalinity is sufficient to neutralize the acid, even if any is secreted. It has been shown on dogs, that any substance such as mustard, which by its irritating qualities will largely increase the secretion of mucus, will to a great extent neutralize any free acid that may be present.

Pepsin and rennin are usually present in chronic gastritis, unless the case is one of long standing. Analysis shows that the proteid elements of food are not changed as much as they should be; meat fibres are generally un-dissolved. Carbo-hydrates may be normally digested, or this process may even be farther advanced than ordinary, because the action of the ptyalin has not been stopped by the gastric contents becoming acid, as normally occurs. At least this digestion of the carbo-hydrates may be thus. unduly hastened, unless they are enclosed in some proteid envelope; as for example is the case in the starchy corpuscles of the cereals. Here the cellulose envelope, if not ruptured by heat before eating, may not be dissolved in the stomach, because of the absence of the hydrochloric acid, and therefore the starch enclosed cannot be acted upon by the ptyalin.

Diagnosis.—To differentiate from ulcer: In gastritis there is not as severe pain immediately after eating; there is no circumscribed spot especially sensitive to pressure, the tenderness being more diffuse; there is no hæmatemesis and there is decreased secretion of hydrochloric acid except in cases mentioned as being sometimes called acid gastritis.

Gastritis differs from cancer of the stomach, in there being less pain, no hæmatemesis, no tumor, no cancerous cachexia. Moreover, in cancer that has advanced to any great extent lactic acid and the Oppler-Boas bacillus are usually present in the stomach contents. However, gastritis is usually associated with cancer, and the diagnostic symptoms of cancer should be carefully looked for before eliminating the possibility of its presence in cases presenting the symptoms of chronic gastritis.

Certain forms of nervous dyspepsia have often been diagnosed as chronic gastritis, especially by those who do not make a practice of analyzing the stomach contents. If sufficient care is taken, this need not often occur, for besides the differences in these contents, in the troubles due to nervous conditions, there are usually other symptoms of a nervous character, and there is a greater variation in the symptoms depending upon mental or emotional conditions.

After a case has been diagnosed as chronic gastritis, it is important to decide whether it is primary, or whether it is secondary to some other trouble, as mentioned under the etiology. This can be done only by examining thoroughly for such conditions, by methods taught in those departments.

Prognosis.—Chronic gastritis, uncomplicated, probably never causes death, but, it may so impair nutrition of the individual that he is more susceptible to other diseases, such as tuberculosis or pernicious anæmia. And these diseases, together with others, either acute or chronic, that may arise, will be much less amenable to treatment, than those in patients possessing a healthy stomach. Although alone it may not be fatal, yet it may be very long lasting, and difficult to relieve. Of course if destruction of the glandular elements has taken place, it is impossible for the stomach to return to a normal condition; yet, careful and long continued treatment, may cause a disappearance of active symptoms, the patient made comparatively comfortable, and a fairly good state of nourishment be maintained. Some cases taken before any destruction of glandular elements has taken place, may be entirely cured.

Treatment.—As prophylactic measures, avoidance of errors and excesses in eating and drinking may be mentioned. The teeth should be kept in good condition, both that they may more perfectly perform mastication and that they may not provide cavities in which bacteria may lodge, multiply and finally pass to the stomach and infect the food and gastric mucosa.

When the condition has developed, of the measures that may be employed for its relief, may be mentioned,—

Lavage.—This is of considerable benefit in some cases, especially those that are accompanied by much mucus, and where there are evidences of considerable fermentation. It may be performed either with plain warm water, or some mild antiseptic, as boric acid, thymol or hydrastis. Nitrate of silver, 1 to 1,000 solution, followed by plain warm water is very useful, especially in cases presenting a good deal of mucus. If, because of excessive mucus, or because the gastric walls have become relaxed and distended it seems difficult to remove all the sticky, adherent contents, it is often advisable to first wash out the stomach with some alkaline solution, as of bi-carbonate of sodium, and follow this with whatever other medicated solution is desired.

Dietetics.—The selection of food depends to a considerable extent upon the intensity of the disease. If it is of considerable severity, it will be best at first to depend upon liquid or semi-liquids, such as barley, rice or oatmeal soups, prepared in milk. Follow in a few days with beef bouillon or chicken soup, with perhaps the addition of an egg or some butter. The amounts taken should be small and frequently repeated, possibly four to six times a day. When the symptoms have somewhat abated, any of the lighter vegetables may be added, such as potatoes mashed in milk, green peas or beans cooked until very soft. When these can be borne without trouble, the diet should be increased and an attempt made to improve nutrition. For this purpose all soft vegetables may be used. The amount of meat should be controlled, as its digestion is slow and imperfect, because the secretion of hydrochloric acid is limited; however, it may be given in fairly liberal amount, if it is properly prepared. Meat should be strictly fresh, and very thoroughly divided, by scraping, chopping, cooking or mastication. It should be thus prepared so that it may easily pass the pylorus where it can be acted upon by the trypsin of the pancreatic juice.

Therapeutics.—

Arsenicum album 6x:—Where symptoms of gastric irritability are pronounced. Nausea and vomiting. Burning pains, dry red tongue, great thirst and anxiety. Stomach apt to have been injured by cold food or drinks, beer or tobacco. Pale face, cold extremities, emaciation, weakness and anæmia.

Argentum nitricum 6x:—Like arsenicum there is apt to be much irritability, but there is more belching of gas and more mucus in the stomach contents if vomited or obtained by stomach tube. Great distention of the stomach. Patient craves sweet things, but if eaten they disagree. Very sensitive to pressure, pain immediately after eating and remaining for a long time. Tongue may be black, with a red streak down the middle, or may be red and dry with papillæ erect. Gaseous distention is a very prominent symptom.

Antimonium crudum 3x:—The most marked symptom is nausea, perhaps with vomiting. There is a thick, milky white coating on the tongue. Much fermentation. Belching, with taste of the food the same as when eaten. Pressure in pit of the stomach. Desire for acids, but no appetite for food.

Bryonia alba. 3x:—There is a white tongue, but the coating instead of being moist and milky, is very dry, and there is much thirst for large quantities of water. Nausea and faintness when sitting up, or upon moving. After eating there is pressure in the pit of the stomach, as if a stone were there. Bowels constipated, stools appear dry and burnt.

Pulsatilla 3x:—Tongue coated yellow, or whitish yellow, especially at posterior portion. Slow digestion with taste of food remaining in the mouth a long time, especially if it be fatty food. Nausea aggravated by smell of food cooking. Loathing and nausea at thought of food. Sour eructations with feeling of weight in stomach. Everything tastes bitter.

Hydrastis 3x:—A very useful remedy where there is much mucus, ropy in character. Poor appetite, weak digestion, especially for bread and vegetables. Dull aching in stomach, causing a weak feeling. Tongue coated yellow, with slimy, sticky fur. As result of trouble extending to duodenum, the bile ducts are apt to be affected, giving rise to some icterus, especially noticeable in the whites of the eyes.

Sulphur, Kali bichromicum, Calcarea carb., Ipecac, Sepia, Tartar emetic, Siliciea, and many other remedies may be useful in some cases, but when these remedies are useful there are generally complications and the case is not one of simple chronic gastritis. For instance, when associated with liver trouble, China, Nux vomica, Mercury, Podophyllum, Lycopodium, Chelidonium or Leptandra may be appropriate; with heart disease, Digitalis, Nux vomica, Arsenicum or Cactus; if occurring with kidney affections, Mercurius corr., Cantharides or Aurum mur. Anæmia or chlorosis, when especially prominent, may call for Ferrum, China, Nux vomica, Pulsatilla, Sulphur or Calcarea carb.

CHAPTER XIV.
GASTRIC AND DUODENAL ULCER.

Inasmuch as ulcers of the duodenum are usually of the first inch or two beyond the pylorus, and due to the same causes as are those of the stomach, the symptoms are so similar and the treatment is practically the same, it seems desirable to consider ulcers of the duodenum at this time in connection with those of the stomach.

Definition:—A circumscribed loss of substance of the mucous membrane. Occasionally they may penetrate to the deeper coats.

Etiology:—The causes of these ulcers have not been satisfactorily demonstrated. Different writers have given different theories. In reality it is probable that no one cause can be given for all cases, but that instead, a number of them exist. According to one author there are three general causes. These are:—

1.—Mechanical and chemical causes.
2.—Interference with the vitality of the tissues.
3.—Bacterial infection.

As examples of mechanical causes may be mentioned ingested fish bones, egg or oyster shells, seeds or other hard substances, and corrosive or irritant poisons. Any of these may so injure some spot of mucous membrane that it undergoes necrosis.

In the second class of causes, the vitality of a part may be diminished by local or constitutional diseases, or by interference with the circulation of the blood to a certain area, as by thrombosis or embolism; and the gastric juice

then exerting its digestive powers upon such partially
devitalized spot, causes destruction of the ulcerated place.
A combination of this method with the third general cause
is probably the most frequent occurrence. That is, a
thrombosis or embolism occurs, plugging up a minute vessel supplying some circumscribed area. This spot then becomes less resistant than normal; then if a focus of bacteria becomes localized here, an inflammation is produced
which so softens the tissues that during the next cycle of
digestion the gastric juice digests a portion of the mucous
membrane, leaving the ulcer. In practically all cases of
ulcer, the gastric juice is richer in hydrochloric acid than
normal, and this fact is thought to be of importance as it
acts more strongly upon any spots, the vitality of which
is lowered. Certain constitutional conditions also seem
to have some influence in producing an ulcer. Such conditions are anæmia, chlorosis, syphilis, tuberculosis, malaria and various other diseases which have a devitalizing
effect upon the walls of the blood vessels.

Pathology:—The typical ulcer is round and looks as
though it were cut out with a punch. If of but recent origin there is but a slight degree of inflammation around it.
If of longer duration there may be an accompanying inflamed base which may become much indurated and result
in pronounced thickening of the stomach wall at this point.
Frequently, instead of being round, the ulcers are irregular in outline. As regards size, they may vary from almost microscopical dimensions, to five or six inches in diameter. As to location, about 85% of those within the
stomach are on either the pyloric sac, or the posterior surface or lesser curvature near the pylorus. Only 15% are
on the anterior surface and cardiac extremity. Of those
on the duodenal side of the pyloric valve, practically all

are in close proximity to that valve. Quite a common location is across the valve, saddle fashion, part of the ulcer being in the stomach and part in the duodenum. Duodenal ulcers are much more common than was thought a few years ago, many cases of so-called indigestion, the etiology of which was not properly understood until quite recently, being due to such an ulcer. The reason that most ulcers are found close to the pylorus, either on the stomach or duodenal side, is probably because the gastric juice gravitates to this area, thus producing its digestive effect on the membrane, and also because the mechanical activities are more pronounced in this location than elsewhere.

The ulcer may heal, leaving a cicatrix which has a tendency to contract. If this occurs near the pylorus, its contraction may cause a constriction of the outlet. If the scar is located farther from the pylorus, possibly near the middle of the stomach, its contraction causes partial division of the cavity of the organ into two parts. This division may become so extreme that only a narrow orifice remains for the passage of food from the cardiac to the pyloric portions. Such a condition is called hour glass stomach. If cicatrization does not take place, the ulcerative process may either continue and cause corrosion of a blood vessel with resulting hæmorrhage, or it may cause perforation of the stomach walls. If this takes place, when the serous coat is reached one of two things may result. There may be a reactive inflammation causing localized peritonitis surrounded by a zone of adhesive inflammation, or there may be perforation into the general peritoneal cavity, with resulting general peritonitis.

Symptomatology:—Usually the first symptoms of gastric ulcer are indigestion, with a sensation of uneasiness or pain at the pit of the stomach. Nausea and vomiting may be present, though these symptoms are frequently absent. This condition may last a long time without either increase or decrease in intensity. Whether the ulcer remains a mild one, or whether it becomes severe, pain is the symptom, which though varying in degree is practically of chief importance. In character, it may be merely a feeling of weight or tightness across the stomach, or it may become of a cutting, boring or lancinating nature. In ulcer of the stomach, it generally comes on immediately after eating, and continues during the period of digestion, or else until the stomach empties itself by vomiting. In ulcer of the duodenum it appears when the food is beginning to pass out of the pylorus; that is one or two hours after eating. In this respect it resembles the distress of hyperchlorhydria, and must be differentiated from this complaint. In ulcer of either place, coarse or indigestible food causes more severe pain than light or liquid foods. When the lesion is in the stomach, the pain is generally located in the median line, a short distance below the ensiform process. When in the duodenum, it theoretically should be a little to the right of the median line, but in reality this difference of location is not always present. At these points, in an area of less than two inches, there is extreme tenderness on pressure. The pain is also apt to be felt in the back, appearing there somewhat later than in the epigastrium. When there, it is generally on a level with the eighth or ninth dorsal vertebra, and often a little to one or the other side of the median line.

If vomiting takes place, it generally appears later than the pain, usually occurring an hour or two after eating; although sometimes it comes on seemingly as soon as food touches the ulcerated area. Instead of vomiting, pyrosis may be present. In either case the ejected matter generally tastes extremely acid. If vomiting continues till the stomach is empty, the pain is then relieved until food is taken again. Ulcer of the duodenum is not as apt to cause vomiting as ulcer in the stomach.

Hæmorrhage, when present, is the most characteristic symptom of gastric ulcer. However, it is a comparatively rare symptom, occurring only when the ulcer has penetrated the walls of a blood vessel. The size of the vessel cannot be determined by the amount of blood ejected in the hæmatemesis, because sometimes only a part of the blood may escape by the mouth, while the rest of it passes into the intestine, and in ulcer of the duodenum the larger part or even all of it may take such course. If the blood is vomited, its color may vary widely, depending upon how long it has remained in the stomach; if but a short time, it will be bright red; if longer it will be darker, or even black and tar-like, as a result of the action of the hydrochloric acid. If, instead of being vomited it passes into the intestine, it comes away in the form of black, tar-like stools. Hæmorrhage may be so severe and sudden, that death occurs before vomiting takes place; in which case the cause of death may be unknown unless an autopsy is · held.

Patients with a gastric or duodenal ulcer are apt to have a good appetite, but owing to the fact that eating causes so much distress, they usually take food very sparingly. As a result of this, and also because of the vomiting, and perhaps hæmatemesis, they are apt to become emaciated and weakened. Constipation is generally present. In women, as a result of the anæmia which is apt to develop, there is sometimes amenorrhœa. In other cases hæmatemesis may occur in the form of a vicarious menstruation.

The gastric contents in practically every case, are characterized by an increased secretion of 'hydrochloric acid. Besides the symptoms already mentioned, others of a less characteristic nature are often found. These may vary to a considerable extent, and they are those indefinite ones that are apt to exist in nearly all cases of so-called dyspepsia. For instance, there is apt to be considerable gas to be expelled, and if the patient is successful in emitting it freely, there will be considerable temporary relief from the pain. A bad taste which is probably due to starchy fermentation sometimes exists, especially in the morning. In fact, as said before, there is always an excessive degree of hydrochloric acid present, and therefore added to the symptoms of ulcer, there are those mentioned under hyperchlorhydria.

Diagnosis:—If hæmatemesis of large quantities of bright red blood exists, it is sufficient upon which to base a diagnosis. Fortunately for the patient, however, this is not frequent, and so the diagnosis has to be made upon less positive signs. The character and time of appearance of the pain are of some help, but in many cases are not sufficient. Other diseases may have pain of a quite similar nature, and the time of appearance varies somewhat depending upon the location of the ulcer. Vomiting is by no means always present, and even if so, it may also be present with numerous other diseases. Examination of the stomach contents is not sufficient basis upon which to form a diagnosis, as the only finding is the same as that found in hyperchlorhydria. The most definite sign is the discovery of a small, circumscribed spot, located as mentioned above, which is extremely tender upon pressure. In eliciting this sign, care must be exercised, as some patients, especially those of a hysterical or neurasthenic type, may appear very sensitive, when in fact there is no organic lesion present. In examining such patients, it is well to engage their attention by some conversation entirely foreign to the subject of pain, at the same time casually pressing on the suspected spot. In doing this with purely nervous cases, they will give no evidence of distress, but if there is an ulcer it is impossible to so distract their attention, that pressure will not produce cringing and other signs of being hurt.

In the history of cases of ulcer of the stomach or duodenum, there is apt to be a marked periodicity. That is, there have been several attacks, of varying lengths of time, during which the epigastric or digestive distress was felt. These spells are followed by other periods of comparative relief. Many times, however, the attacks of suffering have been more severe upon each return, have lasted longer and have been more difficult to relieve, and the periods of feeling well have been correspondingly abbreviated.

Prognosis:—It would seem that no better information can be given, than is found in Einhorn's book on Diseases of the Stomach. He says: "In one hundred cases of ulcer, there were perfect cures in fifty, perforations and peritonitis in thirteen, foudroyant hæmatemesis in five, pulmonary tuberculosis in twenty, inanition in five, and different complications in seven."

In considering the prognosis, it is important to give attention to other affections which it has been shown are apt to come indirectly as a result of ulcer. For instance, it is now recognized more than a few years ago, that where ulcers have continued for a considerable time, and are either still existing, or have healed, leaving scar tissue behind, there is a great tendency toward carcinomatous degeneration developing on such a base. Besides such local danger, ulcer often induces a poor state of nutrition, so that tuberculosis or other constitutional diseases are more liable to develop. Even where such serious conditions do not appear, a gastric or duodenal ulcer has a great tendency to recur. Treatment will generally cause relief of the symptoms at the time, but a slight indiscretion as regards diet or general care is very apt to cause a return of the trouble, so that a patient with this malady often gives a history of attacks similar to the present one coming on repeatedly for a period of several years.

Treatment :—The treatment which has gained the greatest reputation, is the so-called Leube-Ziemmsen cure. This is carried out as follows: The patient is kept in bed for a period of three weeks. Hot poultices are kept on the epigastric region during the day, and at night a Priessnitz is applied. If there has been no hæmorrhage the treatment may be commenced at once. If there has been a recent hæmorrhage, it is better, during the first week to feed exclusively by rectum, after which, during the second week, half a cup of clear milk, of strained barley, oatmeal or rice, plain water or weak tea may be given every hour. The food should be taken very slowly, and be of medium temperature. This diet should generally be continued a week. During the next seven days, give the same foods, but in twice the amount and feed once every two hours. During the next week allow food every three hours, the cereals need not now be strained, and soft boiled eggs, and soft crackers or toast may be taken. At this time the poultices may be stopped, and the patient allowed to be-gin getting up, at first for only a few minutes, lengthening the time a little each day, until by the end of another week he can stay up most of the day. Food in greater variety may also now be taken, and by the end of another week a normal diet, of easily digested foods, free from hard particles may be eaten. In cases where there has been no recent hæmorrhage three weeks of such treatment is genrally sufficient; if there has been such hæmorrhage four weeks had better be taken, and in some cases it may be wise to prolong the treatment for a still longer period. One must judge of this matter by the rapidity with which pain, tenderness and nausea disappear. For a considerable period, at least, one should be careful that only bland and non-irritating foods are taken, and also that no heavy work is performed. During the course of such treatment, the bowels should be kept moving. For this purpose, the regular Leube-Ziemmsen treatment, as carried out by its originators, calls for the use of the Carlsbad Sprudel mineral water. In this country it is customary to use the natural Carlsbad Sprudel salt, which is made by evaporating the spring water. A dose should be given every morning, of sufficient size to produce two or three daily evacuations. Usually a teaspoonful in half a cup of hot water will be sufficient for such purpose. If the gastric juice is highly impregnated with hydrochloric acid, as it generally is, it is well to give some alkali to neutralize such acid. For such purpose half a teaspoonful of bi-carbonate of soda, or the same amount of equal parts of bi-carbonate of soda and calcined magnesia may be given every two hours.

Recently certain German physicians have claimed that gastric ulcers are usually caused, or at least kept from healing, because of anæmia. They have therefore put forward a treatment which differs considerably from the above, their efforts being directed to the building up of the patient and relieving the anæmia. In their treatment, the patient is fed liberally, even immediately after a hæmorrhage. Iced milk in which eggs are beaten up, is the food used at the beginning, given in amounts up to 300 c. c. of the milk, in which three eggs have been beaten. From the third day sugar is allowed, from the sixth day scraped meat, then milk, rice and fine bread, and from the tenth day raw ham and butter. Rest in bed, application of ice and the administration of iron and arsenic complete the treatment. Lenhartz, the author of this form of treatment, claims to have better success than by the older method outlined above. However, others who have employed it have as a rule failed to secure as good results.

By medical treatment the great majority of gastric ulcers can be cured, at least temporarily. It is a fact, however, that a great many return upon the slightest indiscretion in diet or working. Many times they recur repeatedly, and the history of a case is a repetition of attacks for a period of several years. After such a continuance of the trouble, there is apt to be a considerable thickening about the pylorus due to cicatricial tissue, with resulting obstruction to the passage of chyme from the stomach to the intestine. Then the vomiting and other distress is aggravated, and gastric dilatation is a consequence. When this condition has arisen, surgery is applicable. Gastroenterostomy is generally the operation of choice, and in selected cases has given extremely desirable results. It is, however, undoubtedly a fact that in recent years many operations have been done for gastric ulcer, that were unjustified. Present opinion does not justify operating unless there is decided pyloric obstruction, and even then it is better first to give the patient an opportunity for a thorough trial of judicious, and continued medical and dietetic treatment.

Therapeutics:—If there is hæmorrhage, the remedies given under hæmatemesis should be studied. For the ulcer itself,—

Arsenicum alb. 3x.:—Is frequently given. There are the characteristic symptoms of burning, lancinating pains, with nausea and vomiting. Anæmia and emaciation are pronounced. There is apt to be a red and irritable tongue, and food causes immediate distress and nausea.

Argentum nitricum 6x:—In chlorotic cases. Severe pain below the ensiform process, extending through to the back. Much belching of gas. This remedy in the 2x, freshly prepared in distilled water, and given in twenty drop doses in a wine glass of distilled water half an hour before each meal, is a very useful remedy. In milder cases it will often effect a cure without the patient being put to bed, provided sufficient care is at the same time given to the diet.

Kali bichromicum 3x:—Where vomited matter is ropy and tenacious. There is much pain of a boring nature at the pit of the stomach.

Mercurius sol. 3x:—Where the epigastrium is excessively sore and distended. Cannot bear pressure of the clothes. Burning, gnawing pains, worse at night.

Phosphorus 6x:—Obstinate vomiting, especially of water as soon as it gets warm in the stomach. Quite apt to be more or less hæmorrhage.

Bismuth sub-nitrate:—This is often extremely useful, given in teaspoonful doses of the crude drug in half a glass of water, half an hour before eating. It is supposed to form a protective coating over the inside of the stomach, including of course the ulcer, and at the same time has a stimulating effect on granulations in the base of the ulcer. Either this remedy or Nitrate of Silver given as mentioned above have often been used in cases where the patient did not think himself sick enough to go to bed and take the regular Leube-Ziemmsen treatment. If either of these remedies is used persistently enough, giving enough care to the diet and rest, many cases may be cured, although the cure can always be secured more quickly and certainly by the treatment in bed.

If cases that do not respond desirably or permanently to medical treatment, and that give signs of poor drainage from the stomach, were treated by gastroenterostomy, un- doubtedly many could be saved years of semi-invalidism, and some would be prevented from going into states of malnutrition making them susceptible to other constitu- tional diseases. In many other cases cancer of the stomach would be prevented, as it has been determined that such malignant growths in many cases are the result of cellular degeneration of cicatricial tissue resulting from long con- tinued ulcers.

CHAPTER XV.
CANCER OF THE STOMACH.

The stomach is more apt to be affected with cancer, than is any other organ of the body. From one-fourth to one- third of all cancers are found in the stomach.

Etiology:—The same as for cancers in other parts of the body. However, it is thought that cancer is more apt to be found in the stomach, if there has previously been an ulcer present. It seems to develop from the cicatrix left by the ulcer.

Pathology:—Like cancer of other parts, it may be di- vided into four classes:

1.—Epithelioma or adeno-carcinoma, presenting a soft, distinct prominence or tumor, upon the surface of which smaller fungoid elevations develop. Each fungosity contains a loop of blood vessels, giving a red color to the growth. Histologically this form consists of cylindrical epithelial cells, bound together by connective tissue fibres in the typical cancerous manner. After a variable period of time, owing to disturbances of circulation, necrosis takes place, and ulceration results.

2.—Medullary or soft glandular cancers also have fungous projections from the surface, which, owing to the small amount of connective tissue contained, are very soft and spongy. Ulceration occurs early in this form, and hæmorrhage is a prominent symptom. Secondary metastases are very frequent.

3.—Schirrus cancers are characterized by a large amount of connective tissue, and a relatively small number of cells. They are therefore very hard to palpate, and, upon section, appear almost cartilaginous. They have no tumor, but rather simple thickenings of the entire wall. In the early stage, ulceration is rare, but when older, superficial ulcers may form. As a rule they do not cause a very profuse hæmorrhage, but rather an oozing of blood. Secondary metastases are not as marked as in some of the other forms.

4.—In the colloid or mucous carcinoma, the cells contained in the connective tissue alveoli undergo colloid or mucous degeneration. The whole growth then has a gelatinous appearance.

The above forms are not always distinctly separated, but sometimes different kinds are found in the same growth. At other times they may change from one kind to another. The schirrus is most frequent. Out of 183 cases 132 were of this variety, 32 were medullary, 17 were colloid, and 4 were epitheliomata.

Cancers may affect any part of the stomach, but are most frequent near the pylorus. Out of 360 cases, 60% were at the pylorus, 10% were at the cardiac end, and the remaining 30% were scattered over other parts. A gastritis of the entire mucous coat generally exists when there is cancer at any part of the stomach which has progressed to any extent. The lymphatics of the diaphragm, abdominal cavity or other parts are apt to become cancerous as a result of metastases, while surrounding organs as the liver, gall bladder and pancreas, are apt to be involved by contiguity. More distant organs may also be involved, as the uterus, lungs, spleen and intestines.

Symptomatology:—Usually a person in middle life or beyond, having previously either had good health, or else giving a history of ulcer of the stomach, begins to feel uneasy after meals. The appetite becomes poor, sleep disturbed and strength fails. These sensations increase in intensity, and the following symptoms in about the order named develop:

Anorexia,—is apt to be present early, and may become so pronounced that there is an actual aversion to food, especially of an albuminous nature.

Pain,—is a very constant symptom, and is usually of a lancinating nature. The situation of the pain varies, and does not always correspond to the seat of the lesion. It often becomes very severe, and although there may be remissions, there is never complete relief. It is but little or not at all influenced by the taking of food; but if ulceration has taken place on the surface of the growth, then eating may increase the pain decidedly. Although the pain is generally lancinating, it may in some cases be described as dull, gnawing, burning, or be attended by a sense of weight, oppression, tightness or distention.

Vomiting,—is a very frequent symptom, especially when the disease is at the pylorus. It may take place after eating, or be independent of it. When the cancer is located at the pylorus and has reached a point where there is partial obstruction, the vomiting may take on the characteristic of being absent for two or three days, then coming on very profusely, remnants of food that had been eaten at any time since the last vomiting attack being expelled.

Hæmorrhage,—is apt to be present in cases that have undergone ulcerative processes. The blood generally oozes slowly into the cavity of the stomach and lies there an indefinite time mixing with food and the gastric secretions, during which time it undergoes changes so that when expelled it is rather dark colored and granular in appearance and resembles coffee grounds. Sometimes, however, a large blood vessel may be eroded so that blood comes away more profusely and is of a bright red color.

Tumor,—when present in sufficient size to be palpated, constitutes a prominent physical sign of cancer. It usually yields a sense of being hard and irregular in outline, but is sometimes smooth. It may become large enough so that it can be seen. Transillumination by means of the gastro-diaphane may reveal a darkened zone, and by the position of this zone some idea of the location of the tumor may be obtained. Occasionally it is difficult to determine positively whether the enlargement is of the stomach, or whether it is of the gall, bladder, liver or pancreas. If of the stomach, it is more movable than of the other organs, provided adhesions have not formed. Distending the stomach with air will shift its position somewhat. Attention may also be directed to the fact that tumor of the stomach is not always cancer, but may in exceptional cases be a cicatricial thickening which has reached a degree where it can be felt, or a syphilitic gumma. In the latter condition there should be a history of syphilis, and the iodide of potassium in proper doses, instead of irritating the stomach, should relieve the trouble.

Cachexia,—is present in nearly all cases which have progressed far enough. When characteristic, it is evidenced by emaciation, weakness and a sort of dry, straw colored appearance of the skin.

Fever,—is not a regular symptom, but may be present in the later stages. It is probably due to inflammation of surrounding tissues, or to absorption of toxic materials from the growth.

Constipation is generally present, because the pyloric obstruction and frequent vomiting lessen the amount of fæcal matter contained in the intestine. Sometimes it alternates with diarrhœa as a result of an associated enteritis, or this may be due to sloughing of the neoplasm.

The gastric contents in the great majority of cases, show an absence of free hydrochloric acid; and if the process has progressed far enough so that stasis is present from pyloric obstruction, there is usually lactic acid present. Microscopically under the same condition the so-called Oppler-Boas bacillus may be found. The finding of lactic acid in large enough amount to respond to the usual tests employed in its detection, and of the Oppler-Boas bacillus, is practically always diagnostic of cancer of the stomach. However, in cancers of the pylorus which have not progressed sufficiently to cause obstruction, especially if developed on the base of an ulcer, and in cancers located at other points on the stomach wall, these findings may not be present. Therefore it is not safe to wait until these agents can be found in all cases before making a diagnosis, because valuable time will be lost by waiting. In cancer of the cardiac orifice, which has progressed to any extent, it is difficult or impossible to swallow food. It may be retained in the œsophagus for a time, thus distending it, and finally be expelled without having reached the stomach. Attempting to pass a stomach tube will of course also meet with resistance in such cases.

Diagnosis:—Max Einhorn says: "The diagnosis of gastric cancer can be positively made under the following condtions:

1.—"If particles of tumor are found in the wash water, which under the microscope reveal the characteristic picture of cancer.

2.—"The presence of a tumor with uneven surface, belonging to the stomach, and associated with dyspeptic symptoms.

3.—"The presence of a tumor associated with frequent hæmatemeses.

4.—"Constant pains, frequent vomiting, ischochymia, emaciation, all these symptoms quite permanent, and not extending over too long a time. (1 year).

5.—"Tumor and ischochymia.

6.—"Emaciation, ischochymia, presence of lactic acid."

Possibly the second of the above propositions should be modified, for in exceptional cases as said above, syphilitic gummata, located near the pylorus, have been palpable and have caused dyspeptic symptoms. At such times the administration of iodide of potash will clear up the diagnosis. With this exception probably these statements cover all cases in which a positive diagnosis can be made. Patients will sometimes be met with who cannot be placed in any of these classes, and yet who present symptoms that arouse one's suspicions. Sometimes time will show that such suspicions were well grounded.

Prognosis:—Gastric cancer generally results in death within at least eighteen months, but sometimes it will be longer. A few cases have now been reported, in which, when the case was properly diagnosed early enough, and a partial or complete gastrectomy performed, complete cure was produced. In other cases the fatal outcome was postponed for a considerable period.

Treatment:—A nourishing diet, and one easily digested without the aid of hydrochloric acid should be selected. If the orifices are affected, as is usually the case, the diet should be liquid or semi-solid. Therefore broths, soups, gruels, raw or soft boiled eggs, scraped meat and purees of vegetables should be employed. By such means the nutrition should be kept at as high a point as possible while foods can yet pass the obstructed orifices; after this time, and possibly even before, as an assistance, it may be well to employ rectal feeding. Where the pylorus is becoming closed, temporary relief from the vomiting, and some improvement in nourishing the patient may be obtained by doing a gastro-enterostomy. Some benefit may also be had from lavage. Washing out the stagnating and fermenting contents relieves somewhat the irritation present, and will thus reduce the thickening of the mucous membrane covering the growth. Medication may be used in the wash water to assist in performing this shrinking, especially nitrate of silver, 1 to 1,000 solution, or a mild solution of adrenalin. Washing out the stomach, when the patient becomes somewhat used to it, is also much easier than the vomiting which will otherwise be present, and will empty the organ much more completely of its objectionable contents.

Remedies are used chiefly for their influence on the gastritis which is generally associated with the cancer, and for the vomiting and hæmatemesis. Their indications are given under those headings. Before the end occurs, it is generally necessary to resort to morphia hypodermically, or opium suppositories per rectum, for the amelioration of the pain. Despite all that can be done, death from cancer of the stomach causes probably as great and prolonged sufferings, as any from which one may die.

Part III.—The Intestines.

CHAPTER I.

EXAMINATION OF THE FÆCES.

Casual examination of the stools has undoubtedly always been practiced, but their thorough study, macroscopically, microscopically and chemically is a development of recent years. Even at the present time so much attention is not given to such examination, as is given to that of the urine or the contents of the stomach. The reasons for such neglect are various, but the chief of them is undoubtedly the fact that such work is unpleasant to one's æsthetic sense, as well as its being objectionable to the patient to take steps needful for providing the examiner with the necessary sample.

However, much of the unpleasantness may be mitigated by the exercise of certain precautions. The portion of fæces to be examined should be placed in a large-mouthed bottle or fruit jar, and immediately covered with water, —to which, if desired, some aromatic, such as menthol may be added. While making the examination much of the work may be done under the surface of the water, using suitable instruments to select parts desired for microscopical or chemical analysis.

Fæces are examined for two purposes:—

1.—To look for elements indicating pathological lesions, parasites or other foreign substances of the intestine.

2.—To acquire information as regards the process of the digestion of foods as performed in the intestine.

To accomplish the first of these purposes, no especial preparation is necessary as regards a test diet, except when making the analysis for occult blood. The stools should be examined for mucus, blood, pus, epithelial cells, fragments of tissue, bacteria, biliary or pancreatic calculi, and parasites or their ova. In addition, judging from the color or by the employment of Gmelin's test as in urine, a determination as to the secretion or elimination of bile may be made.

Mucus, if present in considerable amount, may generally be seen with the unaided eye. If in smaller, but still abnormal quantity it may be discovered by the microscope. Its presence should be so limited, and its admixture with the fæces so complete, that it cannot be discovered except by careful chemical test. If it is otherwise found it may indicate only an irritation of the mucous glands due to the pressure of a solid stool against a portion of the intestinal wall, or it may indicate a catarrhal process of the lining membrane. In such case if the mucus is intimately mixed with the fæces, it ordinarily shows that the process is located in the small intestine, possibly the upper part of it. On the other hand, if the mucus forms a coating on the outside of the stool, it shows that the catarrh is of the large bowel.

Blood may be seen macroscopically or with the microscope if it comes from the lower part of the bowel. Hæmorrhoids, fissures, severe inflammations or ulcers, may give rise to it in such location. If its origin is higher up, it is usually not discoverable by these methods, because the digestive processes performed in the intestine act upon the corpuscular elements to such an extent as to destroy their identity. Sometimes large hæmorrhages, even from the duodenum or stomach, may be followed by so-called tarry stools, which really consist of blood that has partially undergone digestion. In cases open to such suspicion, however, one should be careful to know whether the patient has taken bismuth or any other drug that may have produced the discoloration. At other times when the hæmorrhage is small, or there is uncertainty as to its presence, it can be detected only by a chemical test for so-called occult blood. Before this test, the patient should have been on a diet free from meat for several days. It should be determined that blood has not been swallowed from bleeding gums, nose or pharynx, and the possibility of pus, or unchanged fatty elements must be eliminated. A large portion of fæces is mixed with one-third its volume of glacial acetic acid to produce a fluidity. Place some of this fluid part in a test tube and shake with ether. After the ether has been allowed to rise to the top, pour it off and mix with ten drops of freshly prepared guaiac tincture(one part of guaiac resin to 25 parts of absolute alcohol). Old oil of turpentine which has been exposed to the air for several weeks by standing in a flat dish, is then added, a drop at a time, shaking after each drop, until 20 or 30 drops are added. A slightly blue tint to the layer of ether, shows the presence of hæmatin, and so indicates blood. In shaking the tube do not cover it with the finger and allow the ether to come in contact with it, for in so doing, if perspiration is present it may cause the blue coloration. If blood is discovered by this test it usually indicates an ulcer of some portion of the gastro_intestinal tract. Of course its further location must be letermined by other means.

Pus may be difficult to discover, even if present. It may be only in isolated portions, and microscopical exam_ination must be depended upon to find it. If it exists in small amounts it probably indicates only an irritation of the mucosa. If in larger amounts, it may have come from an ulcerated area or a ruptured abscess. Like blood, if pus originates in the upper part of the intestinal tract it may be so changed by decomposition or digestion that it is not discoverable in the fæces.

Epithelial cells of all kinds lining the intestine, are normally present to some extent in the fæces, and may be detected by the microscope. If present in larger numbers than ordinary, they indicate an undue exfoliation as a result of some inflammatory or ulcerative process. However, anything definite can seldom be learned from their study.

Fragments of mucous membrane or other tissue may exceptionally be found. Care must be exercised that they be not mistaken for portions of food which have escaped digestion. They are usually from ulcerative or necrotic portions of the intestinal walls, or from hæmorrhoidal or other tumor masses. Their nature should be determined by careful staining and microscopical examination.

The *bacteriology* of fæces is too extensive a subject to consider in a work of this kind. Bacteria are found in great numbers, and in a considerable variety and their study must be left to books on bacteriology.

Parasites and their ova are also better left to works on such subjects. The ones most frequently found in this country are the tænia, ascarides and lumbricoides, although other varieties may be found, especially in other countries.

Biliary and pancreatic calculi can best be discovered by first diluting or mixing the fæces with water, then straining through a rather fine sieve or colander. Their indications, if thus discovered, are self-evident.

In studying the fæces to obtain information in regard to the digestive processes as performed in the intestine, it is quite important to have the patient on a test diet. The object of such diet is to have the three varieties of foods,—protein, fats and carbohydrates, in definite amounts, so as to provide a standard as to what is normal. The test diet usually employed is the one advised by Schmidt of Dresden, and as given by him is as follows:

Morning' 0.5 of a liter of milk and 50 grams of zwieback.

Middle of forenoon: 0.5 of a liter of oat meal gruel (made with 40 grams of oat meal, 10 grams of butter, 200 grams of milk, 300 grams of water and one egg); this should be strained.

Dinner: 125 grams scraped beef broiled slightly, and mixed with 25 grams of butter, 250 grams of mashed potatoes (190 grams of potatoes, 100 grams milk and 10 grams of butter).

Middle of afternoon: Same as in the morning.

Evening: The same as in the middle of the forenoon.

This test diet for the entire day contains 120 grams of albumen, 111 grams of fat and 191 grams of carbohydrates, and furnishes 2,234 calories.

This diet may of course be modified to meet personal idiosyncrasies, or in testing for certain specific purposes, but in ordinary cases it is best to adhere quite closely to it. The patient should be kept upon it for three days, and the dejecta of the last day are suitable for investigation.

A portion of this in a large flat dish is mixed with water until it becomes liquid, during which admixture a macroscopical examination should be made for fragments that appear undigested or otherwise differing from normal. Then a drop or two of the fluid, or any suspicious looking pieces may be examined by the microscope. The search as regards the processes of digestion should be for:

1.—Portions of the food which even a healthy person can not digest. These include largely the cellulose elements of vegetables and connective, elastic and cartilaginous tissues from animal food, as well as hairs or other such indigestible constituents.

2.—Remains of food which can be digested but for some reason have not been. Such remnants may be albuminous, fatty or carbohydrate. In estimating the albumen, chief attention is given to the presence of muscle fibres. If such fibres are found which show their transverse striation, it is considered that their digestion has been below the standard. Occasionally rather small, rounded, non-striated portions of fibres are present even in the healthy. For this reason the prominence of the striation is the distinctive feature. If such fibres are found to any extent, it indicates that some part of albuminous digestion is at fault. It may be gastric and show a lessened secretion of the peptic glands, or it may be pancreatic and show that, owing to disease of this organ, the trypsin is not secreted in proper quantity or degree of activity, or else, owing to some obstruction, it is prevented from reaching the intestine. It is often difficult to determine whether the stomach or the pancreas is at fault, but such decision is helped by also investigating the fat. If this is present in abnormal amounts, it is likely due to pancreatic disease which interferes with proper secretion or elimination of steapsin; provided, of course, it can be shown that bile, which is also necessary for the digestion of fat, is present.

Fat is found in the fæces in different forms. In the healthy adult under the Schmidt diet, it should be found only as unstained flakes, or as yellow calcium crystals. If present in too large amount it may be seen as fatty drops or fatty soaps of earthy alkalies consisting of needle-shaped crystals, sometimes presenting in great numbers. The presence of excessive fat in the stools, when not eaten in too large amount, may indicate disease either of the pancreas or of the liver, or some condition of the intestine which has caused a chemical reaction of its contents that is not of the required degree of alkalinity for the proper activity of the bile and steapsin.

Carbohydrates in the stool are detected by finding the starch granules of varying shapes and sizes, depending upon whether they are from potatoes, wheat or other vegetable foods. Their elucidation may be assisted by the use of iodin, because of the fact that starch turns blue in its presence. A fermentation test is also sometimes employed to determine approximately the quantity of carbohydrate material present. Various forms of apparatus may be employed for this purpose, but perhaps Einhorn's saccharimeter as used for urine is as useful as any. Its employment however, as well as that of various other more or less complex chemical tests for the determination of fatty or albuminous products is unnecessary. The use of these methods is as a rule no more satisfactory than are the microscopical findings, and the tests are much more difficult and tedious to execute. An excess of carbohydrate elements in the fæces only proves that a physiological function is not well performed, but does not show in itself what the anatomical reason is for such failure.

In fact examination of fæces for the purpose of studying digestive processes, is not of itself very definite in its results, yet, to the thorough and careful clinician, when used conjointly with other methods of diagnosis, it may be extremely helpful in some cases.

CHAPTER II.
INTESTINAL DISEASES.
DIARRHŒA.

Definition:—An abnormal frequency of evacuation of fæces, which are thin in consistency. Although but a symptom of some other affection, it is of sufficient importance to merit separate consideration.

Etiology:—It may be the result of either of two intestinal functions being improperly performed:

1.—The fæces may contain too much water because of an excessive secretion and transudation from the glands and vessels of the intestine.

2.—An increased degree of peristalsis may cause such a rapid passage of fæces through the intestine, that there is not opportunity for the usual absorption of the liquid parts.

These abnormalities may be produced by any one of the three general etiological factors, viz:

1.—Where the irritation arises from the intestinal contents.

2.—Where the irritation arises from the nervous system.

3.—Where the irritation arises from the blood.

Intestinal contents which may cause irritation are certain articles of food, such as fruit, cucumbers, turnips, sour milk, etc. They may be purgative medicines, or there may be retention of fæcal matter in some of the valvulæ conniventes or sacculi of the intestine, which undergoing fermentation causes irritation and diarrhœa. Some of the intestinal parasites may also cause irritation of the intestine.

Through the nervous system diarrhœa may be produced:

1.—By anything irritating the nerves causing peristalsis.

2.—By anything paralyzing the nerves inhibiting peristalsis.

3.—By the presence of an increased irritability of the intestinal secretory nerves.

As examples of irritants acting from the blood, may be mentioned the diarrhœa occurring in uræmia, malaria, septicæmia, lithæmia, etc. These poisons being in the blood reach the intestinal glands and excite increased secretion.

Treatment:—If caused by purgative medicines, the diarrhœa will probably subside of itself when they have been eliminated. Parasites or fermenting fæcal masses, or other forms of irritants should be removed. If due to nervous diseases treatment should be directed to their cure. The same can be said where noxious materials in the blood, act as exciting causes.

As to treatment of the symptom itself, if the patient is quite severely affected, he should be put to bed. Even in the milder cases a cure would undoubtedly be more quickly produced if this were done. Externally, warm applications are useful, especially if there is pain.

The diet in diarrhœa is of prime importance; in fact if this is not attended to, the most carefully made prescription will probably fail. In acute cases the amount of food should be lessened temporarily and it is often best to stop food altogether for the first twenty-four hours. Care should then be taken not to give anything likely to undergo fermentation, or that has much of a residue. No fruits or vegetables should be allowed. At first some bland liquid food is best, such as barley water or arrow root gruel. A little later small amounts of mutton broth may be given, and when some progress has been made this may be thickened with a little rice, tapioca, sago or cracker crumbs. In some cases milk, diluted with lime water may be used. As improvement continues, such articles may be allowed as milk toast, oysters, boiled rice, the white part of chicken, baked or mashed potatoes and soft boiled eggs. One should wait until the stools have been normal for some days before returning to the usual miscellaneous diet.

Chronic diarrhœa requires some modification from the above diet, but as it is usually the result of chronic enteritis, its diet will be more fully considered under that heading.

The remedies chiefly useful for the relief of diarrhœa, together with their indications are as follows:

Arsenicum album. 3x:—After chilling the stomach with cold substances. Stools are slimy, with much mucus; offensive; preceded by cutting pains in abdomen. Burning in anus and rectum. Restlessness, thirst, prostration, anxiety. Often useful in chronic diarrhœa. Aggravated by eating and drinking. Often a red irritable tongue; frequently nausea, sometimes vomiting.

Mercurius corrosivus 6x:—Diarrhœa apt to occur in damp weather, or hot days with cold nights. Stools brownish, or green and slimy. May be blood with stool. Usually much desire, with scanty results. Great tenesmus; great desire to strain, without relieving; may be some abdominal colic but most distress is in rectum.

Podophyllum peltatum 6x:—Especially useful in hot weather diarrhœa, and in babies during dentition. The chief characteristic is the changeability of the appearance of the stools. During the course of a few hours they may possess a variety of colors, as yellow, white, brownish and greenish. They may be liquid, lumpy or formed. They are usually frequent and not accompanied by much pain, but may be preceded by some distress of a griping character. Stools smell sour, and are apt to be more frequent in the morning.

Aloes socotrina 3x:—Worse in hot, damp weather; stools yellow and jelly like. Sudden and extreme desire, with inability to control the sphincter ani sufficiently to retain the stool. Much flatulence and gurgling in the abdomen. Aggravated by eating, drinking and in the morning upon rising to the feet, because of the paretic condition of the sphincter.

Croton tiglium 6x:—Stools are copious, yellow, watery and usually painless, although they may be preceded by some sharp, cutting colicky pain in the abdomen. Escape from the rectum suddenly as though shot out of a gun. Desire for stool immediately after eating or drinking.

Colocynthis 3x:—Necessary characteristic is the intense, colicky pain, causing the patient to bend forward, possibly over some hard surface as the edge of a table. Stools are generally copious, fluid, yellow and frothy.

Chamomilla 3x:—Especially in children during dentition. Stools are white and shiny, or yellow like scrambled eggs, with possibly a greenish tint. They are very offensive, smelling like rotten eggs. Colic before or during stool, with relief afterwards. Child is cross; cries and whines constantly. Wants everything it sees, but is not satisfied when it gets it.

Ipecacuanha 3x:—Is also frequently useful in teething children, and in autumn diarrhœas after eating unripe fruits. Principal characteristics are the persistent nausea and vomiting accompanying the diarrhœa and the greenness of the stools. They are as green as grass.

Aethusa 3x:—Only useful when there is an intolerance for milk, which is vomited as curds as soon as taken. Stools are also of curdled milk.

Aconite 3x:—Diarrhœa from catching cold or getting wet; after a suddenly checked perspiration. Also from anger or fright. Stools are apt to be green, scanty and frequent. There is fever, with thirst, and a hard, frequent pulse.

Veratrum album 2x:—Characterized by violence of the symptoms and the sudden and extreme prostration. Hippocratic countenance. The stools are frequent and copious They may be greenish, or yellow, mixed with blood. Also rice water stools. Severe colic, with nausea, vomiting, weakness and shuddering.

Calcarea carbonicum 3x:—Fat, scrofulous children, with fair complexion and open fontanelles. Stools white and chalk like. Appear undigested; at first they are hard and lumpy, then pasty, the last part being liquid. Offensive odor. Sweat on head when sleeping; cold, damp feet.

Sulphur 30x:—Usually chronic diarrhœa, in scrofulous people, although if certain symptoms are present it may be useful in acute form. Early morning diarrhœa driving patient out of bed. Stools are variable in appearance, and smell fetid; the smell seeming to cling to the body. Aversion to washing. Prostration and emaciation.

Belladonna 3x:—More apt to be in children who have diarrhœa as a result of cold. Probably some fever present, and with cerebral symptoms. Considerable colicky pain, relieved by bending backward. Stools are sometimes green; generally contain mucus, and there may be blood.

China 3x:—Accompanied by symptoms of "biliousness." Stool contains food particles and smells putrid. Generally painless and is worse at night, and after eating. There is rapid emaciation and prostration.

Elaterium 6x:—Cutting colicky pain, followed by gushing, frothy stools. Patient is weak and feels cold.

Lachesis 30x:—In extremely low forms of disease, as septicæmia, pyæmia and some forms of typhoid, accompanied by diarrhœa. Stools very offensive and putrid in character. Patient in condition of stupor. Involuntary bowel movements.

Phosphorus 6x:—Prostration with diarrhœa, which may be involuntary. Rectum must empty itself as soon as stool enters it. Diarrhœa is painless and may contain white particles looking like rice.

Rheum 3x:—Colic and tenesmus, followed by slimy, acid stools. Entire patient smells sour. Stools generally brownish and frothy.

Undoubtedly other remedies may be called for in exceptional cases, and no attempt has here been made to give all the symptoms which may be present for consideration in selecting the remedy, but only those symptoms which are most characteristic, and, which, in the majority of cases, are the most prominent ones presenting themselves for relief.

CHAPTER III.

CONSTIPATION AND OBSTIPATION.

Definition:—By constipation is meant a condition of tardy and insufficient fæcal passages, due to a decrease either of secretion or peristalsis of the intestine.

Obstipation refers to a condition in which there is some deformity or contracture in the intestinal canal, or press-

ure from external growths, causing obstruction to the
fæcal passages.

Etiology of Constipation:—In some families there seems
a hereditary tendency to constipation, succeeding genera-
tions being so afflicted. Old people are apt to have difficulties in inducing a free movement of the bowels, due somewhat to decreased intestinal secretion, but more probably
to a lack of exercise. It is also common in children, due
largely to the nature of their diet. Women are more liable
to be constipated than men. Among the causes producing
this may be mentioned, the monthly enlargement of the
uterus which presses upon the rectum, in pregnancy the
same condition existing to an even greater extent, after
parturition the relaxed abdominal muscles, and sometimes
uterine displacements. In addition, women are less inclined to exercise than men, and owing to modesty or other
reasons frequently neglect the call to defæcation until a
paretic condition of the rectum ensues, so that the call is
not so emphatic as prior to such neglect. Occupations
which are of a sedentary nature may be mentioned as another cause. The food eaten is possibly of more importance
than anything else. Concentrated and animal foods give
rise to small residue, and so do not stimulate peristalsis as
do more bulky foods. A small eater is more apt to have
infrequent movements than a more hearty one, although
by eating an excessive amount it may so undergo fermentation that the resulting gas will distend the intestine to such
an extent that peristalsis will not be active. If fluids are
taken in too limited amount, constipation is apt to result.
Certain drugs and medicines may help to induce constipation; prominent among these are the lime salts, lead, opium, tannic acid, alum, etc. Many digestive disorders tend
to make the patient costive; such affections may be of

the stomach, intestine, liver, or pancreas. Chronic diseases of any organ have a tendency to lessen bowel movement, because in such diseases the amount of exercise taken is apt to be insufficient. In cases of insanity as well as in many other affections of the nervous system, organic or functional, the intestinal activities are not performed as they should be.

Etiology of Obstipation:—In children an imperfect absorption of the septum separating the rectum and anus, abnormalities of the sigmoid flexure or colon; or diverti-. culi, may interfere with the passage of the fæces. In later life there may be hypertrophy of Houston's valves, or other malformation in some part of the intestine. Pressure on the transverse colon by a dilated stomach, dragging down of the hepatic flexure by a movable kidney, a relaxed condition of the abdominal walls, or abnormal length of the mesentery or mesocolon, may cause unnatural bends or kinks of the intestine, resulting in obstruction to the fæcal current. In cases where there has been pelvic inflammation as in peritonitis or cellulitis, it frequently happens that bands of adhesion have formed which prevent a normal peristalsis of the colon or sigmoid, or they may be so placed across these parts that obstruction is caused. Fissures or ulcers in the rectum, stone in the bladder, and some forms of urethral disease, may cause spasmodic contraction of the sphincter ani, interfering with free evacuation. Lastly, foreign bodies or tumors and other enlargements in the intestine itself, or pressing upon it from without may cause the condition.

Symptomatology:—The symptoms produced by constipation may be either local or constitutional. The local ones are produced by the retention and pressure of the hardened mass, and may consist of hæmorrhoids, fissures or ulcers of the rectum, or of disturbances of the urinary or genital organs, especially of women.

The constitutional symptoms may in some cases be reflex as a result of pressure or irritation of the mucous membrane or nerves of the intestinal tract, but probably more frequently are due to autointoxication from absorption of toxins developed in the stagnating and putrefying masses. These symptoms will vary a great deal, depending upon the nature of the toxic materials. There are apt to be symptoms of indigestion, with flatulence, lack of appetite, coated tongue and offensive breath. The nervous system is generally affected as evidenced by headache, drowsiness, mental lethargy and restless sleep. There may be palpitation of the heart, dyspnœa, vertigo and disturbances of vision. The other eliminative organs, namely the kidneys, lungs and skin may show symptoms because of the extra work thrown upon them in an effort to eliminate the toxic materials formed in the intestine and absorbed by the blood vessels and lymphatics. The kidneys may become inflamed or irritated, the lungs are more subject to bronchitis and pneumonia, and the skin appears discolored, or is subject to eruptions.

Diagnosis:—This is easy as far as the constipation itself is concerned, but an effort should also be made to discover the cause, and this may carry one into almost any department of medicine.

Treatment:—This resolves itself into,—

1.—An effort to remove the cause of the trouble.

2.—Treatment of the constipation itself.

As it was said, seeking the cause of the condition may carry one into any department of medicine. The treatment of such cause must be considered from an equally broad view, and, as it is really a part of the treatment of

such other disease or condition as gives rise to the constipation, it is not proper to consider it here. In cases of
obstipation surgery is often demanded for the purpose of
incising hypertrophied Houston's valves, liberating adhesions about the appendical region, the gall bladder or elsewhere, removing tumors, dilating strictures and many
other mechanical conditions.

In treating the constipation itself, diet is of great importance. By its regulation, the fluidity of the stools may
be increased or peristalsis may be stimulated. To increase
the fluidity, the blood pressure must be raised, so that the
gastro-enteric glands will secrete more profusely. This
can be done by having the patient drink plentifully of
liquids, or eat foods that consist largely of water. Intestinal peristalsis may be stimulated either by foods containing much residue, as coarse vegetables, by the friction of hard and coarsely ground cereals, as oatmeal,
graham flour or whole wheat flour, or by eating fruits containing many seeds, especially figs; also by other fruits
containing certain organic acids, which act as a stimulant
to intestinal peristalsis.

Judicious exercise, either general in the open air, or
local as by manipulations and actions of the abdominal
muscles, cold tonic baths and massage may be employed.
Electricity, both general to improve the nerve tone, and
local, one electrode attached to a faradic apparatus in the
rectum, the other one on the abdomen may be beneficial.
Another method which has been of much service is the
use of a rectal plug made so that it can be attached to a
vibrator; by fine and rapid vibration a relaxing effect may
thereby be produced upon the sphincter ani, and also
through the sympathetic nervous system the upper intestinal activities may be stimulated. At the same time the

well-known effect of flushing the capillaries of the entire body by dilatation of the sphincter not only increases intestinal secretions, but also improves metabolism and elimination of the whole organism. The formation of a habit of going to stool and making an attempt at the same time each day is of much value. This kept up for a considerable period, taking plenty of time each day whether successful or not, will frequently help wonderfully in overcoming the trouble.

In judiciously selected cases much can be done with the properly indicated remedy. However, most patients demand immediate results and object to waiting until the condition can be relieved by such treatment. Therefore it often becomes advisable to resort to means by which immediate result may be obtained, while waiting for the more lasting effects of homœopathic therapeutics. Of course, cases that are dependent upon such mechanical conditions as flexures, adhesions, pressure by tumor, movable kidney, dilated stomach, retroverted uterus or hypertrophied valves in the rectum, one cannot cure by medication. In such cases surgery is the only thing that offers much hope of giving relief. If, however, the fæces are delayed only because they are too dry in consistency, or because peristalsis is deficient, constitutional remedies will materially help.

Nux vomica 6x:—Especially atonic cases, and in persons leading a sedentary life. They are irritable and cross, have used much coffee and purgative medicine and are sometimes dissipated. There is headache, tongue coated, especially a yellowish coating toward the base, with bad taste in the mouth worse in the morning with flatulence. Ineffectual urging to stool. Constipation and diarrhœa may alternate.

Bryonia 3x :--Where the fæces are especially hard and dry, with no urging to stool. The tongue is dry and coated white. A congested feeling in the head, especially the back of it, with some dizziness, worse upon moving about, or rising from a sitting or stooping posture. Patient is cross and surly. Feeling of a stone in the stomach.

Hydrastis 2x :—Stools are hard and coated with mucus, or may be clay colored. Gastric and hepatic symptoms of this remedy usually present. Especially a sinking feeling in the stomach. Apt to be hæmorrhoids.

Lycopodium 30x :—Contraction of rectum, with ineffectual urging to stool. Small stool with feeling that more remains. Much flatulence.

Opium 30x :—Lessened peristalsis. Stools consist of hard round balls. No inconvenience from large accumulation in rectum. Absolutely no desire to expel.

Sulphur 30x :—Stools scanty and difficult to expel, although there is much urging. Itching and pressure in the rectum. Great tendency to hæmorrhoids. Scrofulous people with the ordinary sulphur characteristics.

Alumina 6x :—Usually there is a dry lower bowel, with hard stool, but even if the stool is soft, the rectum is so inactive that the stool is expelled with difficulty.

Platina 3x :—The bowels are inactive and sluggish. Patient has feeling that they should move, and that stool is in rectum, yet desire to expel is absent. Stools seem sticky and are of consistence of putty. Useful in the constipation apt to arise in travelers, and due to the attention being attracted to other and unusual surroundings.

Plumbum 6x :—Constriction of muscle fibres both of the intestinal and of the abdominal walls interferes with passage of stools. Retraction of abdomen. There is also contraction of sphincter ani and a feeling as if there were a band attached to it lifting it upward into the pelvis. There is urging to stool, and if any passes it is in small round balls.

Sepia 6x:—Constipation in women at menopause. Bowel inactive, with no desire for several days. Apt to be bearing down sensation in pelvis, which makes patient feel as though she did not dare to strain in order to defæcate. When stool does pass it is large and hard.

Silicea 30x:—There is desire for stool, and every thing seems all right until just as it is passing, then the sphincter contracts and forces the stool back into the rectum.

If conditions demand that the bowels be moved quickly, some mechanical means may be employed, or some laxative or cathartic remedy given. An enæma may be used, either of plain water, or with the addition of soap, glycerine or turpentine. If an immediate and free evacuation is especially desired, an enæma consisting of two ounces of sulphate of magnesia, two fluid ounces of glycerine, turpentine one-half fluid ounce and hot water four ounces, is very effective. If laxative medicines are given by the mouth, one should first decide whether it is desired to stimulate peristalsis or to increase intestinal secretion. If the latter, some of the salines, as magnesium sulphate or sodium sulphate may be employed, or the irritable vegetable cathartics, as elaterium, jalap, etc. If it is desired to stimulate peristalsis, cascara sagrada, aloin or podophyllum may be used. Many times some combination of these remedies is given for the purpose of acting on different parts of the intestinal tract, and at the same time to stimulate the flow of bile. A useful combination, is 1/10 grain each of aloin, belladonna, podophyllin and nux vomica. One to three such tablets at night will usually act by the next forenoon. Castor oil, of course, is an old standby,

and for a single occasion is often desirable if the patient
can be induced to stand the disagreeable taste. For children some preparation of rhubarb, such as the syrup, is
an agreeable preparation. In recent years it has been
found that phenolthallein, formerly used only as a chemical reagent, has laxative properties, and because of its
tastelessness it can be prepared in the form of a confection,
and is often a desirable agent to use, especially for children and women. The method of its action is not well understood as yet, but it produces a softened, painless stool,
and is a fairly useful addition to this kind of remedies.
Tablets containing from one to three grains are generally
employed.

CHAPTER IV.
ACUTE CATARRHAL ENTERITIS.

Definition:—An acute inflammation of the mucous
membrane lining the intestine. Acute enteritis is
the most frequent disease of the intestinal tract
and may affect either a portion of the intestine
or its whole length. If it affects only a part, it may be a
duodenitis, jejunitis, ileitis, typhlitis, colitis or proctitis;
or any two or more of these may be combined. The colon
is the part most frequently involved, and is probably always more or less inflamed when any of the other parts
are affected, and sometimes when they are not.

Etiology:—A variety of factors may act as causative
agents, prominent amongst which may be mentioned,—

1.—A number of kinds of bacteria which gain access to
the intestine and cause enteritis, either by direct action,
or by their toxins.

2.—Excessive quantities of food, by undergoing putrefactive processes, may produce toxins of an irritating
quality.

3.—Chemical irritants, as certain drugs and poisons.

4.—Mechanical irritants, as hard fæces, calculi or other foreign bodies.

5.—Excessively cold substances as ice cream or cold drinks, which first start a stomach trouble that later extends to the intestine.

6.—Variations of the temperature. It may be caused by chilling the body.

7.—Autotoxæmia. From various toxic products circulating in the blood.

8.—Secondary enteritis is very apt to occur in many of the infectious diseases, also in affections of the heart, kidneys or liver, in tuberculosis and diabetes. In most other organic diseases of the intestine, such as cancer, volvulus, intussusception and peritonitis, enteritis is apt to be an accompaniment.

Pathology:—There are hyperæmia, swelling and increased secretion. The hyperæmia may be diffuse or circumscribed. It is more pronounced around Peyer's patches, the apices of the valvulæ conniventes and of the villi. The swelling is manifested by thickening of the mucous membrane, due largely to increase in the size of the blood vessels, and by loosening of the epithelium. These epithelial cells may become so loosened that they separate and are cast off, leaving a raw surface which may take on the character of an ulcer. There is also an increase of the tissue elements, owing to a development of many round cells, which thickly permeate the diseased parts. Owing to a large number of white corpuscles which have migrated from the capillaries, the surface of the membrane may take on a grayish color. In the milder cases there is a covering of transparent, tough, glassy mucus, which may be colored by blood or bile. In more severe cases the secretion becomes opaque, owing to the large number of epithelial cells and leucocytes. In the severest cases, the secretion becomes purulent and the capillary blood vessels and the crypts of Lieberkuhn become distended. The muscular and serous layers do not become affected in catarrhal enteritis.

Symptomatology:—Acute enteritis generally manifests itself by a feeling of fullness in the abdomen, colicky pains and diarrhœa. The number of stools may be only two or three a day, or there may be one every few minutes. The first passages contain normal fæcal matter, later they become thinner, and in time are liquid. The first are brown in color. Then they may change to some lighter shade, as gray, yellow or green. They may contain much mucus, and sometimes blood or pus. Microscopically there are particles of undigested food, and also a great number of bacteria and epithelial cells. Outside of the abdominal symptoms there may in light cases be perfect health. At other times there will be weakness, a feeling of dullness, dizziness, nausea, and if the stomach is involved there is vomiting. If the lower part of the colon or the rectum are inflamed, tenesmus will be present. In children, in whom the disease is especially frequent, and also in old people, the above symptoms are apt to be more pronounced. In the majority of cases fever is absent; at other times it may be present, sometimes as high as 104 degrees. Fever is more pronounced in cases that have resulted from infection by bacteria, either pathogenic or those from tainted food. Physical examination occasionally reveals some bloating, and on palpation there is apt to be some tenderness about the umbilicus, and sometimes all over the abdomen. There are quite often gurgling sounds, due to movements of gas and fluids in the intestine.

In order to find the part of the intestine involved, the following points should be noted. In duodenitis there is generally some icterus present, though not marked, and sometimes it may be absent altogether. Jejunitis and ileitis, if not accompanied by colitis are difficult to diagnose, as diarrhœa is generally absent. If the stools are examined, however, they will probably be found to contain particles of undigested food, mucus and an abnormal number of epithelial cells. Indican is also usually to be found in the urine. Acute colitis is determined by tenderness over the course of the colon, and by pain in this region. The stools are thin and contain much mucus. Proctitis is characterized by tenesmus and colicky pains in the left inguinal region. There is almost constant desire to defæcate.

Prognosis:—As a rule this is good when occurring in adults. Recovery generally takes place in from two days to three weeks. In children and old people it is more dangerous, and in children, especially in the summer, quite often causes death.

Treatment:—If the case is at all severe, the patient should be put to bed. If the state of nutrition is good, total abstinence from food for a day or two is of benefit. In children this should generally be done anyhow, especially as regards milk. These two things,—rest and cessation of food, are of vital importance, and alone they will relieve many cases. If symptoms then persist, a very light, bland diet should be instituted, such as barley water, strained oat meal gruel, bouillon, and in grown people, boiled milk, soft toast and possibly soft boiled eggs. Water may be taken in small amounts, but not taken when it is cold. If there is considerable weakness, a little brandy or wine may be added to the water. A return to normal diet should be made very slowly, being guided largely by the symptoms, the number and consistency of the stools and the amount of mucus contained in them.

The remedies and their indications will be those mentioned under the subjects of diarrhœa and dysentery.

CHAPTER V.

CHRONIC ENTERITIS.

Etiology:—The causes are about the same as in the acute form. In fact it is usually a result either of one severe attack of acute enteritis from which recovery was imperfect, or more frequenly of several milder attacks which have so injured the tissues that they are left in a morbid condition. Like the acute form it may either be primary, or secondary to some other diseases, as affections of the lungs, especially tuberculosis, or diseases of the heart, liver or kidneys. It may also be caused by the irritation of intestinal parasites.

Pathology:—Similarly to the acute variety, hyperæmia, swelling and increased secretion are present. However the hyperæmia is of such a variety that the surface appears grayish or brownish in color, instead of red as in the acute form. In cases of long standing there may be spots that are black, due to the escape of blood pigment from the vessels. These vessels are prominent, and frequently more curved than normal. The epithelial cells are partly desquamated, and many of them are undergoing fatty degeneration. More cells than normal are in the interstitial tissues. The glands are sometimes elongated and tortuous, and their necks may become constricted, resulting in a cyst from retained secretions. Polypi may form. The above description applies to the form called hypertrophic. In some long lasting cases this may change to the atrophic *variety* in either one of two ways:

1.—The gland may undergo fatty degeneration and be destroyed.

2.—The inflammatory process may extend to the connective tissue, which then becomes so hypertrophied that it crowds the glands out of existence.

Both the hypertrophic and the atrophic forms often involve the tissues beneath the mucous membrane. As a result of the former, the walls of the intestine may become much thickened, while in the latter they become thinner than normal. Sometimes in chronic enteritis, especially of the tuberculous variety, ulceration takes place. These ulcers may be small and superficial, or become large and so deep that they are called phlegmonous. They may then cause perforation of the intestine, or they may involve a blood vessel and cause hæmmorrhage. If perforation occurs suddenly, it causes peritonitis and death. If it takes place more slowly, then a localized peritonitis develops, resulting in adhesions.

Symptomatology:—In some cases symptoms are absent, or are so slight as to be hardly noticeable. Usually there is a sensation of fullness, with pressure and pain in the abdomen, and borborygmus. These sensations may be more marked a considerable time after eating, or immediately preceding defecation. Owing to the pressure of gases, especially in the transverse colon, there may be asthmatic symptoms, palpitation of the heart, a congested feeling of the head and vertigo. If the enteritis is severe or has lasted some time, the general health may become affected. The patient then becomes weak, emaciated, irritable, melancholic, and as a result of anæmia has cold extremities and a slow, weak pulse. Gastric symptoms such as nausea, anorexia and belching are apt to be present if the small intestine is affected. If the duodenum is involved the process generally extends somewhat to the bile ducts, and as a result, there is apt to be some icterus. Pressure over the abdomen may elicit some tenderness, either diffuse or circumscribed, depending upon the location and extent of the catarrhal process. It will also cause some gurgling sounds, as a result of movement of gases and liquids. Bloating is frequently present. At other times these symptoms, found upon physical examination will all be absent. As regards the evacuations from the bowels, there are four classes:

1.—Where there is constipation. The nerves controlling peristalsis have been so injured by the inflammation that they are weakened. The stools appear almost normal upon inspection, except that they contain more mucus than should be present.

2.—Constipation and diarrhœa may alternate. The fæces are retained until they putrefy, and thus become abnormally irritating. As a result the nerves controlling peristalsis are stimulated, and the stools are expelled in liquid form.

3.—Occasionally there will be one daily evacuation, which is usually unformed and mushy in consistency, and has flakes of mucus mixed with it, and perhaps more undigested food than there should be.

4.—In the last class, there are for months at a time, several daily, diarrhœal evacuations. The stools are apt to contain much mucus, epithelium and undigested food, and are brighter yellow than usual, because of the presence of unchanged bile. In such cases the catarrhal processes are apt to extend over both small and large intestine: as a result, absorption is interfered with, and the amount of fæces is excessive.

Diagnosis:—Mucus, either in the form of shreds or flakes, which is present in such amount as to be perceptible, is all that is necessary for making a diagnosis of catarrhal enteritis. Of course the process may be present in conjunction with some other disease, so this condition should not be diagnosed as existing exclusively, unless all evidence of other diseases is absent.

Prognosis:—Depends upon the intensity of the symptoms, their duration, and the age and constitution of the patient. In infancy and old age, it is a serious disease. The same can be said when tuberculosis, or affections of the heart, liver or kidneys exist. In recent, uncomplicated cases, occurring in the adult, much can be done for its relief.

Treatment:—Hygienic and dietetic measures are of chief importance. The patient should not work too hard, but should have plenty of out door exercise. He should dress warmly, especially over the abdomen. Exposure to cold should be guarded against, also getting wet or being in a damp atmosphere more than necessary. Meals should be taken regularly and in small amounts possibly taking them somewhat more frequently than usual, so that sufficient nourishment is secured to prevent malnutrition. In cases where diarrhœa exists, the following foods should be forbidden; all acid foods or drinks, all kinds of fruits, all coarse vegetables such as cabbage, cauliflower, cucumbers and tomatoes, and coarse bread, as rye or whole wheat, and sweets and pastries. They may have soft boiled eggs, light meats and fish, white bread well baked or toasted, cream soups, bouillon, rice, sago, mashed and baked potatoes in small amount, milk and tea. Neither foods nor drinks should be taken in large amounts, or when cold. If the diarrhœa is quite severe, the patient should be kept in

,bed for a few days on a very rigorous diet of liquids; then as this symptom improves, a return to a more liberal diet may be made, trying to build him up, as much depends upon improving his vitality. It is often difficult to do this, because if enough food is taken to improve nutrition, the enteritis may be aggravated. By watching carefully, however, and keeping just below the amount that will produce an aggravation, yet giving all that can be borne, the anæmia, and general health of the patient will often be improved to such an extent that the catarrhal process will be materially benefited.

When constipation exists, the patient may have any of the foods mentioned under diarrhœa, and in addition fruits, light green vegetables, plenty of cream and larger amounts of carbohydrates, as bread and potatoes. He should avoid bread made from coarse flour, rich gravies, salads and the coarse vegetables.

The remedies for chronic enteritis will be those mentioned for diarrhœa and constipation, with the same indications. In treating a case it is always well to examine the stomach carefully and its ability to properly prepare food for its entrance into the intestine. For if the food is not thus prepared it acts as an irritant to the mucous membrane and helps to keep up the trouble.

CHAPTER VI.

MEMBRANOUS ENTERITIS.

Definition:—A disease characterized by the discharge of mucous or membranous masses from the intestine.

Etiology:—Nearly all cases are found in women, usually between the ages of twenty and forty. The subjects are generaly of a neurotic temperament, but whether this should be considered as cause or effect, is somewhat uncertain. As a very frequently associated condition, may be mentioned ptosis of some of the abdominal organs, such as the stomach, transverse colon and right kidney. There are also apt to be diseases of the uterus or its appendages, and sometimes the so-called uric acid diathesis. These various conditions often seem to act in the capacity of causative agents, and yet sometimes membranous enteritis will exist with no evidence of any of them being present. Whatever the etiology, there are necessarily two elements present. These are:

1.—An excessive secretion of mucus from the intestinal lining of the colon.

2.—A stasis of the fæces in the large intestine.

The excessive secretion may be due to a neurosis of the secretory nerves of the colon, or it may be a result of inflammation of the mucous membrane. It is probably due sometimes to one, and sometimes to the other. The stasis of the colonic contents may be due to anything that will cause constipation or obstipation, and it is in this way undoubtedly that ptoses, adhesions about the uterus or appendix, etc., act as causes. When this stasis occurs, it allows time for the absorption of the water from the excessive mucous secretion, and the condensation on the mucous surface of the thicker, tougher elements,—the so-called mucin.

Pathology:—This is somewhat doubtful. In some cases no changes of a pathological nature can be found. Because of this fact some authors have claimed that the condition is a purely neurotic one. In other cases, there are the characteristic lesions of a hypertrophic inflammation, and because of this some have claimed that its causes are inflammatory. For this reason the names membranous enteritis, or mucous colitis are generally applied to the condition, although they may seem misnomers.

Symptomatology :—There are three principal symptoms:

1.—Attacks of colicky, contractive pains in the intestine.

2.—These attacks are followed by the passage of the characteristic mucous masses, sometimes in the form of a cast of the colon.

3.—Constipation.

In addition there are generally indications of neurasthenia, the patients becoming easily tired, irritable or despondent, with many of the mental symptoms which are so frequently found in neurotic cases. There may be anæmia and emaciation, although sometimes the patient appears well nourished. The appetite is variable, there is much flatulence and considerable distention of both the stomach and intestine. There is apt to be indefinite pain in the back or sides, and insomnia is sometimes present. On physical examination there may be found a red irritable looking lining of the colon as seen through a proctoscope, or it may appear normal. Often a loose right kidney may be found. Sometimes there is a retroverted uterus or evidence of adhesions in the pelvis; Houston's valves may be hypertrophied and the anal sphincter is generally found spasmodically contracted.

Diagnosis:—This is based on finding the membranous masses in the intestinal evacuations. One should be careful however, to depend upon his own observation rather than the description of the patient, because these masses have been confounded with coagulated milk, orange fibres, undigested fascia from food eaten, and intestinal parasites, especially tape worms.

Prognosis:—In rare cases the disease disappears after a *few attacks.* Usually however it runs a chronic course, and is very difficult to entirely eradicate. This disease alone never causes death.

Treatment:—The diet should be the one recommended for constipation, and an especial effort should be made to build up the nutrition to the highest possible point for the purpose of improving the neurasthenic condition. It has been shown that a diet should also be selected that has a good deal of residue, such as the coarse vegetables, as this waste·matter in the colon seems to have a beneficial effect in lessening the amount of mucus secreted, and the painful symptoms are somewhat modified. If the patient is decidedly emaciated, anæmic and neurasthenic, it will probably be well to give the Weir Mitchell rest treatment, with the forced feeding, massage and electricity to improve such condition. Much benefit may often be derived from the use of olive oil injections. The patient is directed, when she retires at night, to assume the knee chest position and inject from four to six ounces of warm olive oil into the bowel, and, if possible, retain it during the night. This has a soothing, healing effect on the mucous lining and glands, and at the same time helps to keep the colon mildly distended and so prevents to some extent the excessive secretion. If there is a decided tendency to a red inflammatory appearance of the mucous lining, it is better to use a one or two per cent. solution of ichthyol made with the olive oil. This treatment should be given every night for a few weeks, then every other night, and finally once a week. In the morning after such an enæma, if there is not easily an independent movement of the bowels, it is well to take an injection of warm water, to which one teaspoonful of bicarbonate of soda, or of powdered borax has been added to the quart of water. Such cases may also be much benefited by treatments at the office. Havin them placed in the knee chest position, by means of the proctoscope and air pressure get the large bowel open as widely and as high up as possible, then spray thoroughly with a one to five per cent. solution of nitrate of silver. If there is a movable kidney, inflamed or adherent appendix, adhered uterus or hypertrophied Houston's valves, it may be necessary to treat these conditions surgically. The mental or neurotic symptoms should be treated according to their indications. The remedies of chief utility are:

Argentum nitricum 6x:—Very melancholic; weak memory; easily tired; large accumulations of gas in the stomach and abdomen. Reddish or greenish stools, consisting of mucous shreds and muco-lymph.

Kali bichromicum 3x:—Thick yellow coating on the tongue, food lies in the stomach like lead. Aching, stitching or dull pains in the hypochondria. Mucous, jelly-like stools, consisting of tough, stringy material.

Nux vomica 3x:—Cross irritable people; troubles brought on by high living. Much distress in the stomach, with feeling of load, and with flatulence. Frequent desire to pass stool, with ineffectual attempt.

Ignatia 3x:—Hysterical women, melancholy and inclined to solitude. Easily tired. Feeling of emptiness in the stomach. Depressed condition.

Nux moschata 3x:—Great sleepiness, with tendency to faint. Absent minded. Increased appetite. Enormous distention of abdomen after each meal. Much rumbling and gurgling of gas. Tendency to looseness of bowels.

Mercurius 3x:—Very sensitive in region of pit of stomach; abdomen distended with gas; stitches in hepatic region. Mucous stools of yellow or bloody color. Characteristic desire for stool, which is not relieved by the evacuation.

CHAPTER VII.

DYSENTERY.

Definition:—A primary, specific colitis.

Etiology:—The causes may be divided into predisposing and exciting. The predisposing are,—

1.—Climate and temperature. In the torrid zone endemic dysentery is present at all times, but especially in the hotter months of the year, and toward autumn when the nights are cold and the days warm.

2.—Injudicious diet, such as food that easily ferments or putrefies.

3.—Improper hygienic surroundings, such as poor drainage, lack of ventilation and general uncleanliness.

The exciting cause of dysentery in most of its forms, and probably in all of them, is some form of micro-organism. The variety is not always the same, and to consider this point it is better to divide the disease into three classes:—

1.—Endemic dysentery. This occurs only in tropical countries, and is caused by the amœba coli. These were first definitely described in 1874 by Lœssel of St. Petersburg and consist of a coarse granular protoplasm, oblong in shape, and varying from 0.02 to 0.05 m. m. in length.

2.—Epidemic dysentery. As regards the variety of bacteria causing this condition, authorities differ, and it is probable that it is not always due to the same organism. A variety of bacilli discovered by Flexner seems to be the cause of dysentery in the Phillipines, and a similar one described by Shiga to be the cause in Japan.

3.—Sporadic dystentery. A great variety of organisms has been assigned as a cause. It is likely that bacteria normally present in the intestine, become pathogenic at times, and assist in causing this form.

Pathology :—In endemic dysentery the process begins as a diffuse, hæmorrhage catarrh of the colon, and in slight cases does not go beyond this stage. In more severe cases ulcers form, which are characterized by a scanty secretion of a purulent exudate. These ulcers may begin in a solitary follicle or in the mucous coat. When in the latter they communicate with the lumen of the intestine by channels, sometimes small, at other times as large as the ulcers themselves. As above said, these ulcers at first are caused by the amœba coli, but being once formed, a great variety of bacteria assists in keeping them open. The ulceration having been established, there are three processes which accompany it: a fibrinous exudate, a diphtheritic-appearing membrane and a hyperplasia of the intestinal mucosa surrounding the ulcer.

The pathology of the epidemic form has two principal stages :

1.—Catarrhal.

2.—The diphtheritic.

In the first stage the mucosa becomes hyperæmic, then inflamed and later ulcerated. The entire membrane is thick, sodden and infiltrated. After this a layer or membrane of either grayish or grayish red mucus covers the surface. This latter is the diphtheritic stage and is the result of three conditions:

1.—Round cell infiltration.

2.—Necrosis of the epithelium covering the membrane.

3.—A fibrinous exudate forming upon the surface.

The pathology of the sporadic form differs somewhat, depending upon the kind of bacteria causing the individual case, but inflammation followed by ulceration is the chief feature usually found.

Symptomatology:—There are certain prodromal symptoms, consisting of a feeling of weight, pressure and distention in the lower abdomen. If the case is to be an intensely severe one, it begins at once with a chill, followed by fever, nausea, vomiting and anorexia. After this the symptoms vary considerably. In some cases they are more due to the inflammatory or catarrhal stage, in others they are more dependent upon the ulcerative process. There may possibly be no fever, at other times it may reach as high a degree as 104° F. The evacuations are small in amount, usually very thin, and may consist of mucus and blood alone, or may contain some fæcal matter. As the case progresses the stools become like meat juice, containing gelatinous lumps. They may consist of pure blood, either bright red, or dark and decomposed. The number of stools varies from four or five a day, up to thirty or more. They are generally accompanied by severe abdominal pains of a griping nature, and with much straining and tenesmus. These pains are relieved temporarily by the stool, but soon return. As the disease progresses and ulceration takes place, there is pus mixed with the mucus and blood. Later when the diphtheritic process is fully developed, pieces of membrane and necrotic intestinal tissue may be found. Such masses may consist of the deposit of infiltrated cells and fibrin that have covered the surface of the intestine, or they may be the lining of the intestine itself. There is apt to be considerable vomiting, much thirst, rapid emaciation and great prostration. The symptoms may run a course of only two or three days and be followed by relief, or they may be more severe, last longer, and yet be followed by recovery. They may cause death, or they may finally pass into a chronic form. In this latter kind, the stools become less frequent, and fæcal matter is mixed with them. The griping pains and tenesmus are partly or entirely relieved, the patient becomes considerably emaciated and anæmic, the skin is rough and dry, the appetite remains impaired and the tongue red and fissured, the patient continuing in this condition of invalidism for a long period; the weakness and anæmia may become more marked, a hectic fever develop with night sweats, dropsy and albuminuria may ensue and death finally take place.

Treatment:—The prophylaxis has to do with avoiding infected drinking water, infected, unwholesome or excessive amounts of food and insufficient clothing and the disinfection of fæcal passages. In the early part of the disease, the diet should be restricted, and should consist only of small amounts of milk, egg albumen, custards, corn starch and arrow root gruel. Alcohol in the form of brandy or champagne is frequently necessary, for both the nutritive and the stimulating effects. When the fever, pain and tenesmus have ceased, the tongue becomes clean and the stool normal in character, then very cautiously more nourishing food should be given. Begin with raw scraped meat, finely minced portions of the white meat of chicken, fish, eggs and purées of some soft vegetable. Cracked ice may be given to relieve the intense thirst that is usually to be found. As the affection is confined to the colon, a great deal of benefit may be obtained by washing this out with some medicated solution. For this purpose quinine in the strength of one part to 2500 of water has been used and shown to be destructive to the parasites present. If there is much ulceration, a solution of boric acid may be used for its cleansing and antiseptic effect, followed by bismuth sub-nitrate suspended in water. A solution of tannin or sulphate of zinc may be useful for the astringent effects.

In more chronic cases nitrate of silver 5 grains to the quart of water may be used. Normal saline solution may be injected and left in the bowel, helping to relieve the thirst and keep up the blood pressure.

Mercurius corrosive 6x:—This is the remedy most frequently useful for dysentery. The stools are frequent, scanty and composed of nothing but mucus, blood and shreds of membrane, accompanied by very distressing, persistent tenesmus, and cutting, colicky pains, with a sense of burning in the rectum after stool.

Aconite 3x:—In the early stage of cases beginning with chill followed by fever; dry skin, thirst, restlessness and the typical stool of dysentery.

Arsenicum album 3x:—Stools of thick, dark, green mucus; they are watery, bloody and very offensive. Much tenesmus and burning in the rectum. Great exhaustion, thirst for small quantities of water, nausea and vomiting. Face pale and sunken; weak and rapid pulse.

Nux vomica 3x:—Cases that have been addicted to alcohol, or have been taking strong diarrhœal mixtures. Constant desire for stool, with but poor results.

Ipecacuanha 3x:—Autumnal dysentery, after eating unripe fruit, vegetables or sour substances. Stools green as grass, fermented, much colic and excessive nausea. This medicine in large doses has been considered by some of the old school, to have just as specific an effect in dysentery as has quinine in malaria. Others have failed to see any such effect.

Colocynth 3x:—Especially useful in the early stages, with the characteristic pain, aggravated by eating and drinking. Abdomen bloated.

Cantharis 2x:—Great tenesmus, which also affects the bladder in the same manner. Stools contain mucus and blood, and look as though the intestine had been scraped.

Aloes 3x:—Cutting pain about the umbilicus. Bloody. jelly-like stool; sphincter feels weak and relaxed.

Other remedies may be useful, especially podophyllum, belladonna, baptisia, capsicum and sulphur.

CHAPTER VIII.

APPENDICITIS.

Definition:—An inflammation of the vermiform appendix. Prior to 1881 inflammatory conditions in the right iliac fossa were called l y various names, such as typhlitis. peri-para- and epityphlitis, iliac abscess, and iliac phlegmon. But in the above mentioned year Dr. Fitz published an article showing that the appendix was the starting point in nearly all conditions of this kind, and that in many cases the disease was confined to this process. Since that time the word appendicitis has almost entirely supplanted all other designations for diseases of this character, especially in this country.

Appendicitis may vary to a great extent in its manifestations as to severity, variety, extent of involvement and otherwise. However, it is customary to divide it into three general classes:

1.—Catarrhal.
2.—Suppurative.
3.—Chronic or recurrent.

CATARRHAL APPENDICITIS.

Etiology:—To an extent, the causes are the same as those acting in other parts of the intestinal tract to produce enteritis. That is they are mechanical or chemical irritation associated with bacterial infection. The vermiform appendix, being a long narrow tube, offers a splendid opportunity for the growth of bacteria after they have once gained access to its cavity. If plugs of mucus, a piece of fæces or some other foreign body enter through the valve of Gerlach it is difficult for the appendix to expel them, and sometimes such foreign bodies have direct influence in helping to start an inflammation. Whether the inflammation becomes only catarrhal, or whether it goes on to suppuration, depends upon a number of circumstances, such for instance as the variety of bacteria, their virulence, the size and position of the appendix, its condition as regards the circulatory and glandular apparatus, and last and probably most important of all the vitality or resisting power of the individual. If he possesses the ability to develop a high degree of phagocytosis, in other words, if he has a high opsonic index to the variety of bacteria acting, the chances are much more favorable that the case may remain catarrhal, than if such powers of self defense do not exist.

Pathology:—Although strictly speaking the catarrhal process, wherever existing, involves only the mucous coat, yet many times the deeper structures of the intestinal tube suffer more or less from associated conditions. This is especially true in affections of the appendix, to such an extent that the pathology of appendicitis, when not proceeding to suppuration, may be divided into four varieties:

1.—Endo-appendicitis. Confined to the mucous and sub-mucous coats.

2.—Parietal appendicitis. Involves also the muscular coats.

3.—Peri-appendicitis. Extends even to the serous coat.

4.—Para-appendicitis. The process involves not only the serous coat of the appendix, but also the same coat of contiguous parts of the intestine, psoas muscle, ovary or other organ with which it may come in contact. It is this latter form that gives rise to those adhesions which are sometimes so difficult to handle in the operation of appendectomy. A plastic exudate is thrown out in such a case, which becomes so organized that the apposing serous surfaces become firmly glued together.

Symptomatology:—In some slight cases there may be no symptoms. Usually, however, the history of such an attack is about as follows. The patient, possibly after a few days of constipation and sometimes of more or less gastric distress, will notice pain of a colicky nature through the abdomen. At first it is general, later seeming to locate more especially in the right iliac region. At the same time there will probably be loss of appetite, coated tongue, more or less fever, possibly nausea or vomiting, thirst and flatulence. Such symptoms may last but a few hours, or may continue longer, possibly becoming more severe until the patient can scarcely endure the pain. At any time the damage done may be of such an extent that suppuration or gangrene may ensue. To consider the symptoms more in detail:

The constipation may in the first place be due to anything that would cause it under other circumstance. After the inflammation becomes marked there is a rigidity, or many times a marked swelling not only of the appendix but also of the cæcum, which, causing a thickening of the walls, mechanically interferes with the passage of the fæces. As a result of such coprastasis, gas accumulates above the obstruction, causing tympanitis.

The pain is generally the most prominent symptom. At first it is apt to be general over the entire abdomen, or especially in the epigastric region. Later its intensity is localized at the point of junction of the appendix with the cæcum. In a person of average size, this is at the so-called McBurney's point, and on the surface of the abdomen is on a line drawn from the umbilicus to the superior angle of the right ilium, and one and one-half inches from the ilium. At this point there is also much tenderness on pressure, and if the case is a severe one and there are thin abdominal walls a resistance can often be felt, on palpation, which consists of the swollen cæcum and appendix. This examination by palpation, and the finding of the tenderness and swelling is an important point in the diagnosis, and should be carefully done. Care is necessary in eliciting the tenderness, because instead of being in the appendix it may be in the ovary, in a displaced right kidney or in the abdominal muscle itself. At other times it may to a marked extent be only in the patient's mind. In these days there seems to be among the laity a great fear of appendicitis. As a result, any pain in the abdomen immediately causes anxiety, and since most people have at least a vague idea as to the location of the appendix, imagination will sometimes have a good deal to do in leading them to believe that there is pain and tenderness at that point. Therefore while making the examination, it is well to engage the patient in conversation so as to lead his mind into other channels, while casually making palpation over suspected spots. As a result of the tender appendix, the right rectus muscle is always found in a state of rigidity. This spasmodic contraction but adds to the pain. The nausea and vomiting, if present, may be due partly to stagnation of the intestinal contents, and partly to the pain and general distress. The fever varies to a marked extent. In some it may be entirely absent, even in quite severe cases. In others mild attacks will produce marked fever. It is apt to be higher in children than in adults. The urine is generally scanty, high colored. and if constipation is marked it may contain indican. The patient's appearance is apt to indicate a marked degree of distress and anxiety. There is restlessness, but movement only serves to increase the pain. The easiest position is generally on the back with the thighs flexed on the abdomen. These symptoms may continue for only a day or two. or may last for several days, depending considerably upon their severity. and upon the care and treatment which are given to the patient.

Diagnosis:—The above symptoms, especially the pain and tenderness at McBurney's point. should always lead one to think of appendicitis. In so doing, however, one should not forget that other conditions may closely simulate this one; also, that these symptoms are sometimes masked or replaced by others less characteristic. In making a diagnosis it is always extremely important to decide with certainty whether it is of the catarrhal form, or whether it is suppurative. This matter, as well as others pertaining to the question of diagnosis, will be more fully entered into when considering the suppurative form.

Prognosis:—So long as the disease remains catarrhal, and that only, there is no danger to life, although conditions such as adhesions may be forming, which will cause more or less trouble for a protracted period of time. However, since suppurative and gangrenous appendicitis always begin as catarrhal, and since it is many times extremely difficult to determine for a certainty that these forms are not developing, or are not already present, it is better to be guarded in the prognosis.

Treatment:—As soon as the disease is diagnosed, the patient should be put to bed, and all food and drink absolutely forbidden. If there is any vomiting it is best to perform lavage. Quiet and rest should be enjoined. If the patient is restless from pain or other distress, it is best to give a hypodermic of morphia. This not only helps to give rest, but also has a tendency to reduce peristaltic movements of the intestines, and it is certainly best to try to prevent bowel movements for a few days at least. It is partly for this purpose that food and liquids are withdrawn. For the first twenty-four hours at least, it is safer to take absolutely nothing into the stomach except the medicine. After this time, it may be safe to give liquids, preferably water, in small amounts, merely a spoonful or two at intervals of one or two hours. The length of time that it is necessary to be thus careful about taking nourishment depends upon the severity of the case as evidenced by the symptoms. In most cases where one is certain that the condition has not progressed to the suppurative stage, it is best to wait until fever has disappeared, and pain or tenderness are absent, even when not under the influence of opiates. In the majority of cases, this condition of affairs will appear in from three to five days, provided rest and other care and treatment have been thorough. At this time it will be safe to give a teaspoonful of some meat broth or of some strained gruel, three or four times a day. If a day of this causes no exacerbation of symptoms, it will be well the next day to cause a bowel movement. For this purpose there is nothing better or safer than castor oil. From this time on, extreme care must be exercised in the gradual return to a more liberal diet, increasing but slightly each day the amount of food given, and in its change to a more solid form. Very slight haste in doing this will often cause a relapse. The same may be said about too early an attempt to get about, or to perform any exercise. Applications over the painful area are of service, although there is some difference of opinion as to whether it is better to use cold or warm applications. At present probably the weight of opinion favors the use of ice bags, at least duing the first day or two. After this time hot applications seem to be of more benefit. Flax seed poultices are probably as satisfactory as any thing, and will often help to give much relief from the pain. They should be used quite hot, but not so hot as to damage the skin, and cause an open, superficial sore as is sometimes done. Every case of catarrhal appendicitis is the possible beginning of an appendicular abscess that may need operating upon, and if so it is far better to have a healthy skin surface.

The remedies of chief importance in catarrhal appen-- dicitis, are,—

Belladonna 3x:—For its well known indications consisting of flushed face, throbbing arteries, glistening eyes, and headache. The patients complain much of the pain, and there is extreme tenderness upon palpation.

Bryonia 3x:—Sharp lancinating pains, aggravated by motion. There is much thirst, dry, white coated tongue and dizzy headache. The patient seems more collapsed, and presents more of a typhoidal condition than in belladonna.

Rhus tox. 3x:—May be useful where the patient is restless, frequently shifting his position in spite of the pain. An irritable, red, cracked tongue. Indications that the disease is merging into the suppurative form.

Colocynth 2x:—This is more often indicated in conditions of a neuralgic character, but it is also often useful in inflammatory diseases where the characteristic colicky pains are present, causing the patient to bend double.

If all cases of appendicitis in the acute form were secured early enough to be placed upon the above treatment, rigidly executed, but few of them would progress to the suppurative form, and of those which did do so the majority of them would present a circumscribed abscess that could be operated upon and drained in comparative safety. However, many cases are not secured early enough, or for some reason the treatment is not carried out carefully enough. Without doubt even if neither of these features obtains, a certain number of cases will progress beyond a catarrhal form. At such times, operation is often demanded during an attack. It certainly is a fact that one who has had one attack of this disease, is more liable to future attacks, any one of which may become serious. For this reason, especially after the second, it seems the part of wisdom to advise surgical removal of the appendix during ' an interval. At this time it can be done with almost absolute safety; at least the risk of the operation is less than the risk of future attacks.

CHAPTER IX.

SUPPURATIVE APPENDICITIS.

Definition:—In this variety pus forms; it may be as a circumscribed abscess, or as diffuse, purulent peritonitis. Other structures in the neighborhood of the appendix are generally involved, as the cæcum, peritoneum and connective tissue of the right iliac fossa; but as the appendix is in the majority of cases the starting point, it gives the name to the trouble, although it has been shown that in from 5% to 8% of cases the trouble originates at some other point.

Etiology:—It generally begins as a catarrhal appendicitis, and then either because the pathogenetic bacteria are especially virulent, because they find a suitable soil, or for some other reason the disease develops to such an extreme degree that the catarrhal process changes into suppuration.

As there is no way of determining which cases are liable to terminate in this serious form, it is quite important to treat every case of appendicitis as carefully as possible, at the same time watching for the first signs of suppuration. A great variety of bacteria have been found in this condition. The bacillus coli communis is practically always present, but that this alone is not sufficient to cause the condition is evident from the fact that it is often present in healthy appendices.

Pathology:—When the appendix is the starting place, pus generally appears first in its cavity. The accumulation of pus may become so large, or the walls of the appendix so diseased that a perforation occurs and the pus escapes outward. As to the future course, much depends upon circumstances. Possibly preceding the perforation, a circumscribed peritonitis had developed, resulting in adhesions of the appendix to other organs at the point of perforation. More likely a larger area of peritonitis had included a localied zone enclosing the appendix, the cæcum, and various other structures in this locality. When the rupture takes place the pus goes on accumulating, but, being surrounded by this zone of adhesions, the general peritoneal cavity is not affected and the abscess remains a strictly localized one. On the other hand, if sufficient adhesions have not formed, the pus when it escapes is in the general peritoneal cavity, resulting in its entire infection. Another condition which may occur is one where perforation of the walls of the appendix does not take place, but such a severe grade of inflammation develops on the serous coat, that pus is formed and then either the circumscribed or a diffuse purulent peritonitis develops from this starting point. If a localized abscess is formed, its location depends upon the position of the appendix, the direction which the escaping pus takes and the manner in which the adhesions have formed. The abscess may be located anteriorly, posteriorly, internally, externally against the psoas muscle, it may burrow downward into the pelvis or upward toward the kidney. Occasionally the pus, instead of escaping into the peritoneal cavity, may, owing to the adhesion of the appendix to some other portion of the intestine, perforate into it, and thus pass away without further trouble. By the same process, it may escape into the bladder, uterus or vagina, or make its way through the diaphragm into the liver, pericardium or pleural cavity, or through the psoas muscle. However, such terminations are extremely rare.

In considering the pathology of appendicitis, mention should also be made of the fact that sometimes, instead of a suppurative process developing, there is a shutting off of the blood supply to the organ, when a resulting gangrene ensues. This is not only a very serious termination, but it is also extremely difficult to diagnose. Often in this complication, the symptoms are comparatively mild, and not such as to arouse suspicion, until after very serious consequences have resulted.

Symptomatology:—In the earlier part of the attack, the symptoms are those of the condition which then exists, namely, catarrhal appendicitis. These have been described in the preceding article. In typical cases, as pus begins to form the symptoms become more severe. That is, the temperature rises to a higher point, and may become more irregular. The pain becomes more severe, and a greater effort is made not to move because of the added distress. The pulse becomes more rapid, and may be more wiry and smaller. The countenance of the patient takes on an appearance of a more serious condition, becoming somewhat pinched and paler. The right rectus muscle draws up more rigidly. On palpation, especially if the pus is localized and points anteriorly, a more marked tumor may be felt, which can be sharply defined about its margins, or is gradually lost in the surroundings. The skin covering it is movable, but the tumor itself is firmly fixed. If perforation occurs without adhesions having formed, a condition of shock immediately develops, with the characteristic signs of collapse and weakness accompanying. If the seriousness is progressive, a sort of stupor may appear; on the other hand, if the limiting adhesions become firm, preventing extension, or to any extent absorption of the pus products, the condition may improve to a considerable extent. Temperature will then decrease somewhat, although it seldom disappears entirely, the pulse will improve, the appetite partially returns, vomiting ceases, and the distress decidedly decreases.

Although in characteristic cases the formation of pus may be determined by giving close attention to these various details, yet the disease is notably one whose symptoms are not always characteristic. Therefore cases will sometimes be found in which a most painstaking attempt at diagnosis will fail to reveal the true condition. The greater the care that is exercised, the fewer will be such mistakes.

Diagnosis:—Other diseases which have been confused with appendicitis are so numerous that space cannot be given to differentiate all of them. Mistakes in diagnosing the following have been reported: Cancer of the cæcum, intussusception, psoas abscess, floating kidney, typhoid fever, pyosalpinx, fibroid tumor, extra uterine pregnancy, renal abscess, tumors of the kidney, ovarian cyst, dysmenorrhœ, renal colic, pyonephrosis, inflammation of the ureter, dysentery, splenic abscess, tubercular peritonitis, hepatic abscess, rupture of the gall bladder, cholelithiasis, cholecystitis, inguinal hernia, enlarged mesenteric glands, abscess of the abdominal wall, aneurysm of the iliac artery, hip joint disease, lumbar abscess, pneumonia, pleurisy, hysteria and possibly other conditions.

In the majority of cases when difficulty is met, it will be in determining between the catarrhal and the suppurative forms, or rather to determine when the former merges into the latter. In typical cases it should be shown by an increased severity of the important symptoms. That is, there is an increased pulse rate, a higher temperature, more severe pain and an appearance of the countenance possibly merging on the Hippocratic, which indicates a greater degree of suffering and shock. However there are a great many atypical cases, where one cannot be guided by these indications. At such times much help may be obtained by examinations of the blood. A few years ago an increased leucocytosis was thought to indicate pus formation, but later it was shown such is not always the case. However, if a differential count shows that the polynuclear cells have increased out of proportion to the other white cells, for instance if the polynuclears are present in the proportion of 80 per cent. or more of the total count of white cells, pus is generally forming. If a case can be watched by means of this blood count, frequently made, it is of material benefit.

Prognosis:—All depends upon whether the pus is confined by surrounding adhesions, whether there are no such adhesions, or, if present, whether they are too frail to withstand the pressure of the increasing amount of pus. In the first condition careful operation and drainage will save the great majority of patients. In either of the two latter conditions operations are much more difficult, and less frequently successful.

Treatment :—Every case of appendicitis should be carefully treated as outlined under the catarrhal form. If this is done, by far fewer of them will progress to pus formation, and of those which do so advance, more of them will be satisfactorily guarded by adhesions. If in spite of such treatment the symptoms mentioned above as indicating pus, begin to develop, the following remedies are generally applicable.

Mercurius sol. 3x :—A marked tumor, with evidences of suppuration; considerable perspiration; tongue red and dry, or white and flabby. Alternately hot and cold.

Lachesis 30x :—Extreme sensitiveness to pressure; worse when waking from sleep; some delirium; extreme prostration; gangrenous symptoms.

Hepar sulphur, silicea, sulphur and arsenicum may any of them be indicated by the symptoms which characterize these remedies. However, suppurative appendicitis is commonly recognized as a surgical condition rather than one amenable to remedies. As to the best time for operative interference, careful judgment should be employed. As a rule, if appearances indicate that adhesions have formed, it is better to wait until they have become firm, and the active inflammatory process has somewhat subsided. On the other hand if the symptoms are progressive, or shock and symptoms of severity develop indicating the initiation of a diffuse peritonitis, or the rupture of adhesions or of the appendix into the general peritoneum, then the sooner an operation can be done, the greater are the chances for draining successfully.

CHAPTER X.

CHRONIC OR RECURRENT APPENDICITIS.

By this is meant a condition where there have been one or more attacks, very often so mild in character that they were not recognized, which have left the appendix in a pathological state. There may be thickening of some of its coats, stricture of some portion of its lumen, kinking, or adhesions. Associated with such pathology there may be present at all times more or less severe symptoms. These may be local, in the form of pain or distress of some kind, or they may be of a more general nature, and manifest themselves by indigestion, nervousness, constipation and a generally unsatisfactory state of health. There are apt to be attacks when the distress is aggravated, in reality exacerbations of the dormant lesions.

Cases of this kind may last for a long time, and be the cause of much suffering, the origin of which is frequently undiscovered; but generally careful examination will show the nature of the trouble. There is undue tenderness at McBurney's point and sometimes thorough palpation will detect the thickened and hardened appendix. Care as regards diet, exercise and general conduct of one's life will often modify the symptoms somewhat, but for the securing of complete relief, operative measures are generally necessary.

CHAPTER XI.

INTESTINAL ULCER.

Ulcer of the duodenum, as regards etiology, symptomatology and treatment, so closely resembles ulcer of the stomach that sufficient reference has been made to it when considering gastric ulcer. Similar lesions of other portions of the small intestine are extremely rare, except when occurring as a part of some constitutional disease, notably typhoid fever, tuberculosis and syphilis. In such cases it seems more appropriate to study them in works devoted to these diseases.

Ulcers of the large intestine are of more frequent occurrence, especially those involving the sigmoid flexure and the rectum. As books upon rectal diseases give consideration to such ulcers, they will be but briefly described in this article. Some mention should be made of them, however, because of certain symptoms, especially diarrhœa, which are likely to be present and which may be wrongly attributed to other conditions unless one is on the lookout for this malady.

Different varieties of ulcers are found in the lower intestinal tract, the chief of them being,—

1.—Catarrhal.
2.—Syphilitic.
3.—Tubercular.
4.—Toxic.

Catarrhal ulcers may be associated with either the acute or chronic forms of colitis and proctitis. When of the chronic form they are more apt to occur with the hypertrophic than with the atrophic catarrhs. They may be seen either as a single ulcer, irregular in outline, with a base which is red or grayish in color, and which will often bleed easily upon touching it, or be multiple, perhaps smaller, more superficial, and really described more aptly by the term, erosions. If in the rectum or lower sigmoid, they may be easily inspected through a cylindrical speculum or proctoscope. Where indications point to a possibility of such lesions, such examination should be made.

Syphilitic ulcers may look quite similar to catarrhal ones, but usually there seems a greater tendency to thickening around the margins, and a less marked and diffuse redness of the surrounding mucous membrane. Often, however, the differentiation must be made by the history of the case, and by the response to anti-syphilitic treatment.

Tubercular ulcers in the great majority of cases are secondary to tuberculosis of some other part of the body, especially of the lungs, although sometimes tuberculosis of the intestine may be primary. In appearance these ulcers can generally be differentiated by the fact that their edges are more sharply defined than those of the other varieties, and give the impression that they are undermined.

Toxic ulcers may be due to various poisons circulating in the blood. As examples may be mentioned those found in nephritis and diabetes. They are generally multiple and superficial.

Symptomatology:—Ulcers of the upper part of the rectum and of the colon do not as a rule cause any marked pain. Sometimes there may be a noticeable colicky sensation just before stool, in other cases no distress whatever. Diarrhœa is generally a prominent symptom. Sometimes there is nothing characteristic about it, and unless one is on his guard the condition may pass unrecognized. At other times there may be a tendency toward bowel movement especially prominent in the morning when first rising to an erect position. This symptom persisting for any length of time should always induce the physician to examine thoroughly, with a good light through a proctoscope. The stools are generally thin, and if examined will be found to contain some mucus; almost always pus is present, and frequently there are small shreds of tissue and blood corpuscles. The blood may be only in small amount, or it may be so profuse as to be considered a hæmorrhage. General symptoms may be more or less pronounced. For instance, owing to an associated inflammatory zone, there may occasionally be slight fever, especially toward evening, after a day of activity. Often there is an associated nervous condition, the patient being irritable and peevish. If the trouble is confined to the large bowel, the upper intestinal tract may give no evidence of being affected. Sometimes the appetite is good, at other times a bad taste is present, interfering with relish for food. Anæmia and emaciation are generally present, especially after the trouble has lasted for a considerable time.

Diagnosis:—When of the intestine above the sigmoid, ulcers can be detected only by the general symptoms, and the evidences found upon examining the stools. When of the sigmoid or rectum, inspection by means of a suitable instrument will reveal them. At the same time the characteristics of the different varieties as mentioned above may be determined.

Prognosis:—Generally favorable if carefully treated, except of course when tubercular or due to some other severe form of constitutional disease.

Treatment:—Rest in the recumbent position adds very materially to the success of treatment. A diet should be selected which does not leave very much residue to pass over the ulcerated surface; at the same time, especially where anæmia and emaciation have developed, the diet should be nutritious. Nitrogenous foods answer both of these requirements. Milk, koumiss, tender meats, fish, eggs, together with soft vegetables and fine cereals may be employed.

Local treatment is of very material benefit. The patient lying on the left side, with pillow under the hips, should have the bowel irrigated once a day with some cleansing solution, such as the saline or weak boric acid. If there is a considerable tendency to diarrhœa with mucus, pus and even blood, it is well to finish the irrigation with some astringent preparation, such as a 5% solution of fluid extract of krameria, or fluid extract of hydrastis one-half ounce to the quart of warm water, 5 to 10 grains of nitrate of silver to the quart is very useful in stubborn cases. Another good method is to apply powders directly to the ulcerated surface by means of insufflation through the proctoscope. Bismuth subnitrate, orthoform, aristonine, zinc oxide, or zinc stearate may be thus employed. If there is but a single ulcer present, and this can be isolated and reached by application directly through the proctoscope, an application of a 3% or even stronger solution of argentum nitrate may be made to stimulate granulation. Or the solid stick may be carefully used with much benefit to produce a cauterizing effect. The actual cautery is sometimes employed for the same purpose.

The therapeutics of ulcer of the intestine will be covered in general by the remedies and indications given under the subject of diarrhœa. The constitutional symptoms should be given especial consideration in selecting a remedy, as an ulcerated area will heal much more promptly if anæmia or other forms of malnutrition are remedied.

CHAPTER XII.

TUMORS OF THE INTESTINE.

Benign tumors of the intestine are comparatively rare, although adenoma, myoma, lipoma and angioma are occasionally found. They are usually very small, and most often have a pedicle so as to form a polypus, but sometimes possess a broad base. Eighty per cent. of these tumors are found in the rectum.

Symptomatology:—If located in the small intestine such growths do not often cause any symptoms, but may in exceptional instances become large enough to cause obstruction, and they sometimes give rise to hæmorrhage. If in the rectum, they are still more apt to bleed and cause occlusion; and if low enough to be in the grip of the sphincter, they may give rise to tenesmus.

CANCER.

Malignant growths are more apt to be found in the intestine than are the benign. In 6,287 cases of cancer, there were 254 in the intestine.

Pathology:—The adeno-carcinoma is the form which occurs with the greatest frequency, although in the rectum the colloid and the pavement celled epithelioma are sometimes found. Cancer of the bowel is generally primary, very rarely resulting by metastasis from other organs. Sometimes it occurs as an extension from some contiguous organ, especially the stomach, gall bladder, liver, pancreas and uterus. They are found more frequently in the lower part of the intestine. In one hundred and ten cases, six were in the small bowel, seven in the cæcum, nineteen in the transverse colon, and seventy-eight in the sigmoid and rectum.

Such growths usually extend around the lumen of the gut in such a manner as to cause a stricture or a stenosis. If this is marked the intestine above this point becomes dilated, is apt to be catarrhal, and sometimes ulcerates. The cancer starting as it does in the mucous coat, often extends into the muscular and sometimes into the serous. If the serous coat does become involved, a degree of inflammation arises which causes adhesions to surrounding structures. When the growth ulcerates, as it does in the later stages, it may only be on the mucous side, or it may extend through the wall, causing perforation, provided adhesions have not formed in advance; if they have so formed, the ulcerative process may extend to the surrounding organs, causing fistulæ into their lumen. Such fistulæ may be into the stomach from the transverse colon, into the bladder, uterus or vagina from the rectum, or through the abdominal wall to the external surface. In case such fistulæ develop, fæcal matter may pass through these artificial openings.

Symptomatology:—General symptoms are similar to those of cancer elsewhere, namely, pain, emaciation, anæmia and cachexia. There is also loss of appetite and perhaps symptoms of indigestion. When much progress has been made, there is more or less obstruction to the passage of the intestinal contents. If there is extension to the serous coat, there may be sufficient peritonitis to cause some fever. The bowel movements are apt to vary. Constipation will exist for some time, causing distention of the bowel above the obstruction. This may persist until means have been employed to move the stagnating mass, or the irritation from the putrefaction which develops may cause a degree of enteritis with mucous secretion so that diarrhœa will ensue. After such free evacuation another cycle of constipation will occur.

When ulceration has commenced, there is apt to be more or less bleeding. It may be only enough to color the stools in patches, or if a vessel becomes eroded a profuse hæmorrhage may take place| Sometimes the stools present evidences of passing a strictured point; especially if the growth is low down. They may be flattened or ribbon-shaped, or pass away as hard balls. Such characteristics are not proof of cancer, however, as they may be found in other conditions.

Diagnosis:—A positive diagnosis can be made only by the finding of a tumor, or as may rarely happen, by the finding of a portion of the growth in the stools. If the upper abdomen be the seat of trouble, the discovery of a tumor is often difficult, and even when found one can not always be sure that it is cancer of the intestine; but, if associated with cachexia, emaciation, occlusion, and is hard and nodular to the touch, it is probably a cancer of the bowel. If the lower part of the rectum is the seat of the lesion, it may be felt by digital examination. If located higher up in the rectum or in the beginning of the sigmoid, it may be seen through a Kelly proctoscope.

Prognosis:—If left to itself, death of course always follows. The length of time elapsing before such an occurrence varies widely. Sometimes cancer of the intestine will be present for several years. Ordinarily it runs a more rapid course, and causes death within a year or two from hæmorrhage, peritonitis, extension to other organs, ileus or auto-intoxication.

Treatment:—If a diagnosis is made before extension to other structures, or glandular involvement, surgical extirpation may be attempted, and if complete may effect a cure. After more progress has been made, palliation may result from the making of an artificial anus, or by an entero-enterostomy. Medical treatment may also be of some benefit, for instance in the advising of a diet which will cause no more irritation to the growth than necessary, but which will keep up as good a state of nutrition as can be done. Attention should also be given to keeping the bowels open by the use of laxatives or enemata. An associated enteritis may be benefited by the remedies or local applications mentioned under these subjects. Lastly, pain must be relieved, as much as possible by the indicated remedy, warm cataplasms or baths, but finally when these fail, by opium or morphia,. administered either by suppository or hypodermically.

CHAPTER XIII.

INTESTINAL OBSTRUCTION.

Occlusion of the lumen of the intestine may come on suddenly, a condition called ileus, or it may develop gradually. Sudden or acute ileus may be due to any one of the following conditions:

1.—Adhesive bands.

2.—Meckel's diverticulum.

3.—Hernia.

4.—Foreign bodies.

5.—Volvulus.

6.—Intussusception.

An adhesive band resulting from previous inflammation of the peritoneum, may be so located that a loop of intestine gets beneath it, and obstruction is caused by compression; or, a longer false ligament may become knotted in such a manner as to entangle the intestine within its grasp. The knot may then tighten to such an extent as to cause a firm constriction around the intestine.

Meckel's diverticulum, which results from an incomplete obliteration of the vitelline duct, may act in a manner similar to such adhesive bands. As a rule this diverticulum is attached by one end to the intestine about three feet above the ileo-cæcal valve. It is about three inches long and the other extremity is generally free, but may be attached to the umbilicus or to the abdominal wall.

Hernia may cause intestinal obstruction. Not only the well known forms of strangulated inguinal and femoral, but also a hernia through slits or apertures in the mesentery or omentum. The intestine may project a loop through the foramen of Winslow.

The foreign bodies which may lodge at some part of the bowel and suddenly prevent the passage of the contents are numerous. An accumulation of fæcal matter may act in this manner, although this is more apt to act in causing the chronic form. Other substances are gall stones, enteroliths, parasites, a Murphy button, or articles which have been swallowed, as stones, marbles, coins, buttons, false teeth or fruit stones.

Volvulus is a twisting of the bowel upon its axis, or into some position so that its caliber becomes occluded. It generally occurs in the sigmoid flexure, although it may happen in the cæcum, ascending colon or the small intestine. The ordinary cause of this condition is chronic constipation. The retained fæces accumulate in the bowel, so distending it that the walls become paralyzed. At the same time, the increased weight drags on the mesocolon. A loop is thus formed which hangs down into the pelvis; then from some change in the position of the body or of the intestine alone, the twist takes place and the ileus results.

Intussusception is the telescoping of one part of the bowel into an immediately adjoining portion. A transverse section of the intestine will show six layers of tissue. Externally is found the segment of bowel into which the intussusception has taken place. This layer is called the intussuscipiens, sheath or receiving layer. Next to this is the so-called returning layer, and inside of this is the entering layer. The two latter taken together are called the intussusceptum. At the point where the returning layer joins the intussuscipiens there is usually a constricted portion called the neck. These various layers are so arranged that mucous coats are in apposition, as are also the serous or peritoneal coats. If the condition continues any length of time, a fibrinous exudate is thrown out from the adjoining serous layers and this soon becomes organized so as to cause adhesions.

Intussusception may occur at any part of the intestinal tract, but the most common point is for an invagination of the ileum into the colon. The length of the intussusceptum may vary from an inch or less up to several feet.

The causes are various, and many times no appreciable reason for its taking place can be discovered. Diarrhœa, dysentery, typhoid fever, whooping cough and other acute diseases have sometimes seemed to have some influence in producing the condition.

In acute intestinal obstruction, no matter what form or what its origin, the intestine above the part occluded differs materially from that below. The former is distended with gas and offensive fæces, while the lower portion is empty and contracted. In the earlier stages peristalsis is very active above the obstruction; later a paralytic condition is apt to supervene. The mucous lining near the occlusion becomes inflamed. Quite often ulcers form, which may end in perforation with resulting peritonitis. The circulation in the intestinal walls becomes much impaired, causing turgescence and darkness of color. If the condition continues, gangrene may develop.

Symptomatology:—No matter what form of obstruction is present, the symptoms are quite similar in many respects. Sometimes there is a history of intestinal disturbances which have lasted a few days. At other times without any warning the real symptoms resulting from the ileus are manifest. These symptoms in the usual order of their occurrence are,—

1.—Pain.
2.—Eructation.
3.—Vomiting.
4.—Meteorism.
5.—Constipation.
6.—General symptoms.

Pain is the first symptom noticed. When the seat of trouble is in the large intestine, the beginning of the pain may be at that point. In a few hours, however, no matter where the occlusion is located, the suffering is in the umbilical region or has become general throughout the abdomen. The pain is due partly to the damage done to the bowel, mesentery and peritoneum, partly to the increased peristalsis which is generally present above the ileus. In the late stages the pain may be lessened or entirely absent. This is due to peristaltic paresis, to a deadening of the sensibilities of the patient, or possibly to the fact that gangrene is present. The severity of the pain varies a great deal, depending upon the amount of gut and mesentery involved, the rapidity of the onset and the excitability of the patient. In the beginning the pain may be somewhat relieved by pressure, but as soon as the peritoneum becomes involved to any extent there is great tenderness.

Eructations are generally present. At first they may give temporary relief, but soon they fail to do so.

Vomiting appears in most cases within a short time, but if the stomach was empty at the time of attack, this symptom may be delayed. When appearing early, it is reflex in origin; later the strong peristaltic movements probably have some influence in producing the symptom. At first, the contents of the stomach are evacuated, then if the condition is not relieved, the intestinal contents and finally fæcal matter are expelled. The explanation of this is that matter has a tendency to escape in the direction of least resistance when placed under pressure. In this case the intestine above the obstruction is distended with fæces and gas. When they are compressed by the diaphragm and abdominal muscles, as in the act of vomiting, the fæces are driven upward into the stomach and then are ejected from the mouth. Ordinarily real putrefactive fæces are not supposed to exist until the colon is reached but when onward progress is completely stopped putrefaction occurs in the small intestine. For this reason, fæcal matter may be vomited not only when the obstruction is in the colon, but also when in the ileum and sometimes even when in the jejunum.

Meteorism is due to an excessive amount of gas caused by the putrefactive processes going on in the stagnant intestine, and to the fact that the absorption of such gas is diminished owing to the condition of the mucous membrane. When meteorism first appears it may give some idea as to the location of the obstruction, by being present only in that region. Later it becomes more diffuse. If the occlusion is in the large bowel, the portion between the point of obstruction and the ileo-cæcal valve becomes greatly distended. In time, the integrity of the valve is overcome so that the gas passes upward into the small intestine. If the trouble has continued for some time, the intestinal walls are paralyzed and the abdomen becomes enormously distended. As the musculature of the walls weakens the resistance is lessened, and the accumulation of gas may thus go on even more rapidly. At this time the abdomen becomes so rounded in shape that it has been referred to as being "barrel shaped". The diaphragm is pushed upward interfering with respiration and circulation, and the stomach, liver, bladder and large vessels of the abdomen are compressed to such an extent that their functions are much impaired.

Constipation is nearly always present. Sometimes bowel movements may continue for a time either spontaneously or by means of an enema, discharging the faecal matter that was located below the occlusion. Exceptionally a degree of enteritis may develop in the lower bowel sufficient to cause a continuation of the passage of mucous stools. In cases of intussusception there is likely to be more or less haemorrhage and rectal tenesmus. The passage of gas by the rectum is absolutely stopped, being permitted only when the obstruction is relieved.

General symptoms, such as shock and collapse, develop as a result of damage done to the peritoneum and splanchnic nerves. There is apt to be a pale surface, cold sweat and a small, rapid pulse. There is dyspnoea and often hiccough. When peritonitis arises, there is fever. Sometimes a serous effusion, resulting from the inflamed peritoneum, adds to the abdominal distention. If the case is not relieved, it goes on until the shock and collapse terminate in delirium, coma and finally death.

Diagnosis:—Three points are of importance in the diagnosis,—

1.—To determine the fact that there is an obstruction.

2.—To determine its location.

3.—To recognize what form of obstruction exists.

If all the above described symptoms were present the diagnosis of intestinal obstruction would be a comparative_ly *easy* matter, but sometimes they are not all to be found, or at least are delayed in making their appearance. Fæcal vomiting is probably the chief symptom from a diagnostic standpoint, yet that may not exist for the first two or three days. On the other hand, this is sometimes to be found in cases of intestinal paralysis, arising perhaps after some injury to the abdomen, or after the release of a temporarily incarcerated hernia.

Atypical cases of general peritonitis, coming for instance from an appendicitis, may offer a picture very closely simulating acute ileus. In typical cases, the two troubles differ in the following features. In peritonitis the fever starts early. in occlusion not until after at least one or two days. In peritonitis, there is great tenderness on pressure. In obstruction, during the early stage, pressure often gives relief. Vomiting of fæcal matter is rare in peritonitis, never early in the disease. In peritonitis, the abdomen at once becomes tense. In obstruction it is at first soft and gradually distends with gas, which is generally first perceived just above the seat of trouble. In peritonitis, after a short time, percussion may demonstrate the presence of effusion. In obstruction, this is not present unless peritonitis also develops.

Extremely severe cases of acute enteritis, and biliary and renal colic may simulate intestinal obstruction to some extent. Generally, attention to the points of chief diagnostic value as mentioned in these various troubles will suffice for differentiation.

Determining the location of the obstruction is of extreme importance, especially if operative interference is contemplated. Such determination applies both to the location with reference to the abdominal wall, so that one may know where to make the incision, and also to the portion of the intestine involved. Occasionally, especially in cases of intussusception into the large bowel, a digital examination of the rectum may detect the apex of the intussusceptum. Examination of the various openings through which a hernia may protrude will sometimes locate an obstruction of this variety. Examination by the vagina might discover a tumor which was compressing the intestine. Palpation of the abdomen may detect a sausage-shaped tumor at some point, especially in an intussusception. If the abdominal parieties are thin, peristaltic waves may be seen, suddenly terminating at some fixed point, which would probably be the seat of the trouble. A coil of intestine may become so distended and tympanitic that its outline may be determined, by either palpation or percussion. Finally the point where the pain is first noticed is of diagnostic import.

In obstruction of the small intestine the important symptoms, such as vomiting—especially of intestinal matter, and the collapse, occur earlier than when the obstruction is located in the large bowel. If located above Vater's papilla, the symptoms are the same as of acute dilatation of the stomach from obstruction at the pylorus. If in the duodenum below Vater's papilla, or in the upper part of the jejunum, large amounts of pure bile will be vomited. If lower down in the small intestine the urine shows indican at an early stage, while if the obstruction is in the large bowel this may not appear at all, or at least not for several days.

If the trouble is in the large intestine, vomiting may be absent. If present, it will not be manifested at so early a stage, especially fæcal vomiting. Meteorism is more pronounced, and will be confined to the course of the colon until the ileo-cæcal valve is overcome. Injections of water may be made into the colon with the idea of estimating the distance of the obstruction from the anus by the amount of water which can be injected and retained, or air may be introduced by an atomizer bulb, and then by percussion the colon may be outlined to the seat of obstruction.

Determination of the form of obstruction may be very difficult, and is sometimes impossible. At other times it is a comparatively simple matter. Close attention should be given to the symptoms and signs mentioned when considering the different varieties, and then logical conclusions which will suggest themselves should be drawn therefrom.

Prognosis:—This is dependent upon the type of ileus present. When due to impaction of fæces, or to the existence of some foreign body, it is comparatively favorable. Volvulus and intussusception may possibly, though rarely, undergo spontaneous cure, or respond to medical treatment. Incarceration by adhesive bands or Meckel's diverticulum is the most unfavorable condition.

Recovery is much more frequent if diagnosis is made early and the case operated, than if allowed to continue until complications have developed.

Treatment:—Medical treatment should have but a limited field in the treatment of acute intestinal ileus. In most cases it should consist only in preparing the patient for operation. In a few cases, if one can be certain that the obstruction is caused by a foreign body, especially when due to fæcal accumulation, efforts to increase peristalsis may effect cure. Volvulus and intussusception have also been reported cured by medical means, but the chances of success are so few, and their application together with waiting to see if they will succeed increases to such an extent the likelihood of serious complications, that it is generally folly to employ such methods.

If there is much vomiting, especially fæcal in nature, lavage will make the patient more comfortable. Sometimes by such relief and by the reduced intra-abdominal tension produced, intussusception of the small intestine may be relieved. Lavage of the colon by removing putrefactive materials located below the obstruction will also be of some avail. Cases of intussusception. of the colon have been reported cured by putting warm water into the bowel under considerable pressure. The process however is not devoid of danger, and is so infrequently successful that it should rarely be employed; certainly not unless the patient is prepared for operation and is under an anæsthetic. If desired, it may then be attempted, and if not at once successful, operation should immediately proceed.

Another measure which should be employed until operation may be done, is to have the patient absolutely refrain from taking either food or drink. Complete rest in bed should be enjoined. Often the pain is so great that morphia should be given hypodermically. At such a time it not only relieves pain but also acts as a stimulant to the heart and lessens peristalsis and vomiting. By so doing the tendency to shock and collapse is not so great.

The surgical procedures which are applicable depend largely upon the form of obstruction present, and are more appropriately considered in surgical works. If performed early, the operation may often be completed at the one seance. If the case has continued for some time it is better, at first, simply to do an enterostomy. This allows the accumulated fæces and gas above the obstruction to escape. The patient is given time to recover from collapse, auto-intoxication and other complications and then the operation may be completed.

CHAPTER XIV.

CHRONIC INTESTINAL OBSTRUCTION.

A slowly developing interference with the passage of the intestinal current. It may be due to the following conditions:—

1.—Fæcal accumulation.

2.—Chronic intussusception.

3.—Strictures.

4.—Neoplasms.

Fæcal accumulation is generally found in patients who have had constipation for a long time. They have possibly been in the habit of allowing the bowels to go several days without a movement. In such a case instead of there finally being an evacuation, either voluntary or induced, the condition remains. It is more frequent in the aged and in the insane. Women, on account of their greater tendency to constipation, are more often affected than are men.

Symptomatology:—General symptoms such as loss of appetite, bad taste, fetid breath, headache, vertigo and general prostration come on gradually. They are undoubtedly due to the absorption of putrefactive materials from the intestinal contents. From the same cause there is apt to be an unhealthy appearance of the skin. It becomes dry and darkened, sometimes eruptions appearing, and there may be slight jaundice.

The abdomen becomes distended by the accumulation, and also by the gas that forms. As a result of the latter, flatulence and eructations are generally present. The sigmoid, hepatic flexure and the cæcum are most prone to these accumulations. Pressure by the mass upon the lumbar or sacral nerves may give rise to pain, which may be

reflected to the genital organs or legs. Colicky pains of a
mild degree may be felt in various parts of the abdomen.
Having reached a point where these symptoms are present,
any one of three terminations may occur:—

1.—Putrefactive processes in the accumulation may
cause such a softening that it is spontaneously evacuated.
The same thing may be induced by the irritating properties
of certain of the toxins developed by the putrefaction increasing the peristalsis.

2.—The entire mass may not be evacuated, but the center of it will become softened by putrefaction or laxatives,
so that a channel is formed, leaving a tube of hardened
fæces in contact with the circumference of the bowel. If
this happens the symptoms will be modified somewhat, as
gas and liquid fæces may pass through the tubular channel and so out of the bowel.

3.—The mass may go on accumulating with no tendency
to recovery. In such a case the symptoms mentioned go
on increasing in intensity.

An intussusception is much more apt to take place suddenly in the manner described under the subject of acute
ileus. Occasionally, however, it comes on slowly, without
at first giving rise to any symptoms that attract attention.
More or less pain finally appears. This pain is paroxysmal
in character, lasting a few minutes, or several hours. There
is afterwards either remission in its intensity, or complete
cessation. The paroxysms may occur several times a day,
or days and possibly weeks may intervene. The intervals
generally have a tendency to become shorter as the intussusception advances. Vomiting may be present, although it
is rare. The bowel movements vary. They may be normal, there may be diarrhœa, or constipation may exist. The
two latter conditions are quite apt to alternate. Blood and

mucus are sometimes in the stool, and after its passage there is often tenesmus.

Strictures in the rectum are nearly always within two inches of the anus, although they may be found in the sigmoid, the colon or even the small intestine. They are generally caused by the contraction of a cicatrix which has followed an ulcer. The clamp and cautery operation for hæmorrhoids will also cause the trouble unless the clamp is put on longitudinally with the bowel. Simple, syphilitic and tubercular ulcers of the colon frequently terminate in stricture. Typhoid ulcers of the ileum have terminated in stricture, although this is extremely rare.

Constipation gradually increasing in severity is the first and chief symptom resulting from a stricture. Then there will be the signs of auto-intoxication, such as anorexia, headache, nervous irritability and melancholia. Later a catarrhal enteritis often arises above the stricture. The constipation may then alternate with diarrhœa. Mucus and possibly blood will be present in the stools.

New growths which cause a gradually progressive intestinal obstruction may be either of the bowel itself or of some surrounding part so situated that pressure is exerted upon the bowel. Tumors of the intestine and their symptoms are described in another chapter. Obstruction resulting from growths of other organs is generally of secondary importance to the primary condition, although attention may be necessary to keep the obstructed bowel from adding its symptoms to those of the other trouble.

Diagnosis:—An increasing tendency to constipation with periods of temporary total inability to effect movements associated with attacks of colicky pain, is sufficient reason to cause one to suspect some form of chronic intestinal obstruction. If there finally develops a complete obstruction, the symptoms are milder than in the acute variety. Symptoms of collapse are absent or at least slight in intensity. Vomiting is but rarely present. Pain, although present, is not of the intensity that it is in acute ileus.

It is of extreme importance to decide as to what gives rise to the obstruction. In fæcal accumulation, it is almost always possible to find a tumor by palpation. It is generally hard and irregular, and it seems possible to change its shape by firm pressure. Usually it is not tender. In most cases it can be reduced in size or entirely removed by thorough irrigation of the colon.

In chronic intussusception, a tumor which is hard and sausage shaped may be found. If located low down its apex may be discovered by rectal examination. There is more apt to be tenesmus, blood and mucus than in any of the other forms.

As strictures in the vast majority of cases are located near the anus, they may generally be found by digital examination. The rare cases located higher up in the bowel offer considerable difficulty in diagnosis, which may be impossible.

Neoplasms large enough to cause obstruction may generally be found by physical examination.

Treatment :—This depends upon the type of obstruction causing the trouble. In chronic constipation, an effort should be made to prevent the condition going on to fæcal accumulation. If it does develop, an attempt should be made to remove the impacted mass. Enemata are generally sufficient for this purpose. In giving them, better results will be obtained by having the patient in the knee chest position. Then through a small rectal tip allow the solution to enter the bowel rather slowly. The enema may consist of soap and warm water, or a tablespoonful of glyc-

erine to the pint of water. Warm olive oil, four to eight
ounces slowly injected and allowed to remain for some time.
will sometimes assist in softening the hard mass. For the
purpose of both softening the fæces and at the same time
stimulating peristalsis, a solution composed of magnesia
sulphate two ounces, glycerine two fluid ounces, turpentine
one-half fluid ounce and hot water four ounces is often
useful when other enemata have failed. In some cases the
accumulation will be so low down and so hard that better
results will be obtained by placing the patient under an
anæsthetic, dilating the sphincter ani and scooping out the
offending mass. If the obstruction is beyond the reach of
enemata or instrumentation, laxatives or cathartics may be
useful. Castor oil is as satisfactory as anything that can
be used. The salines, as magnesia sulphate, sodium sulphate or Hunjadi water, may also be employed. These
agents however, the same as the vegetable laxatives are
more apt to be of service in cases of chronic constipation
to prevent the impaction, than after it has taken place.

Chronic intussusception, like the acute form, is largely
surgical in its treatment. Some relief from its symptoms
may be obtained by giving a light or liquid diet, which,
with massage, and mild laxatives or enemata may keep the
fæces soft enough to easily pass the obstructed point.

In strictures, attention should be given to the diet and
general care. If the strictures are located at their usual
point in the rectum, they may be benefited a great deal by
dilatation. This is best accomplished by using graduated
Wale's bougies. If the strictures are above the rectum,
operative measures may be necessary. They may possibly
be removed by some device of plastic surgery, by excising
the portion of gut containing them and rejoining the ends

of the bowel by end to end anastomosis, or a lateral entero-anastomosis may be done.

Obstruction due to neoplasms, either of the intestine it-self, or those exerting their influence on the bowel by press-ure, is almost entirely surgical in treatment, although of course temporary attention to diet and other precautions may be employed.

CHAPTER XV.

INTESTINAL PARASITES.

The parasites infesting the human intestine, may be di-vided into three classes:—

1.—Cestodes, or tape-like worms.
2.—Nematodes, or round worms.
3.—Trematodes, or fluke-like worms.

Of the cestodes, the varieties called the echinococcus, the bothriocephalus latus and the tænia, are the most impor-tant. The two former varieties are very rare in the United States. The echinococcus is frequently found in Iceland and other countries where the people live in close relation-ship with their dogs. The excreta from an infected dog, gaining access to food or drink, or in some other way be-ing taken into the mouth of an individual, passes to the intestine, and there develops to a certain stage. It then passes through the intestinal wall and migrates to some distant part of the body. No organ or tissue is exempt, but the liver is most frequently infested. The most com-mon result is a cyst which may attain great size. It varies in formation, sometimes being unilocular, sometimes multi-locular, at other times granular.

The indication of the presence of such a cyst, is a very gradual enlargement in the hepatic region. It is gener-ally painless and not attended by fever unless suppuration occurs. By puncture of such a cyst, a fluid may be obtained which under the microscope shows small hooklets which come from the parasite. In this country, echinococcus cysts of the liver are very rare, one writer saying that but 61 cases have been thus far reported.

The bothriocephalus is also rare in this country, but comparatively common in some of the European countries, especially Switzerland, Italy and Russia. In the ova of this parasite there develops an embryo which may enter the intestine of a fish and migrate to the muscle. Then, if the fish is eaten without thorough cooking, this embryo upon reaching the intestine fastens on the mucous membrane and develops into the full grown worm. This may reach a length of fifty feet, and contain as many as 4,000 segments. Its symptoms are severe, its host often being attacked by extreme pernicious anæmia.

The tænia are the most frequently found variety of cestodes, especially in this country. They are divided into several different kinds, but the only ones of interest in the United States are the tænia solium and the tænia saginata.

The tænia solium, or pork tape worm, is a white ribbon-like worm, consisting of a head, neck and body. The head is round and of the size of a pin's head. The neck is thin, not more than an inch long and not jointed. If full grown, the body may contain as many as 350 sections or pro-glottides, as they are called. Those near the neck are very short and narrow, but increase in size for a distance of three feet. Then for several feet they remain practically the same size,—possibly an inch long, and nearly as wide, and toward the extremity farthest removed from the head, again become narrower and shorter. New sections are constantly being formed to take the place of those being cast off. The mature pro-glottides possess both male and female sexual organs,—that is they are hermaphroditic. In the middle of each segment lies the uterus, consisting of a canal with six or eight branch canals extending out like the branches of a tree. On one or the other side, irregularly alternating, is a prominence, from which is an opening, the so-called sexual pore. In the upper part of the segment are the male sexual organs, consisting of small glistening testicles.

A segment of this parasite may become detached from the rest of it and pass away with the fæces. Then, if such segments gain access to the food, or drink of hogs, the ova upon reaching the stomach, lose their capsule and are liberated. They are then absorbed by the stomach or intestine, and entering the circulation are carried to various parts of the body, especially the muscles. Here they develop in the course of two or three months into cyst worms or so-called cystercerci. Microscopically they appear as small, coiled worms. They retain their vitality from three to six years. If such meat is eaten without being thoroughly cooked, the capsule surrounding these cystercerci will be digested in the stomach, liberating a head and neck which have been formed. These pass into the intestine, and from them full grown worms develop.

The tænia saginata, or beef tape worm differs in appearance from the tænia sodium. It is longer, sometimes becoming sixty feet in length. The segments are thicker, stouter and broader. The head is 2.5 m. m. broad, and is flat. It has four powerful suckers, around which there is collected black pigment. The neck is shorter than the pork worm. The side canals from the uterus are more numerous. The method of infection is the same as for the tænia solium, except that it is obtained from beef instead of pork.

Symptomatology:—A tape worm may give rise to no symptoms, or they may become very marked. If present, they vary to a great extent, and may simulate almost any form of digestive disease. Bulimia, is probably more frequently present than any other one symptom, although sometimes anorexia exists instead. Bad taste in the mouth, coated tongue, flatulence and pain of a griping nature may or may not be present.

Diagnosis:—A diagnosis can be made with certainty, only when segments are found in the stools.

Prognosis:—This is favorable. The tænia solium is the more difficult to get rid of, but persistence will generally succeed. It is also the one most seldom found in this country.

Treatment:—Prophylaxis has to deal with the care that food and drink given to hogs and cattle be not infected, with inspection of the meat for cystercerci, and with thorough cooking of the meat before eating.

The curative treatment may be considered as preparatory, the giving of the drug and the mechanical removal of the worm.

The object of preparatory treatment is to have the intestinal tract empty enough so that the remedy used may act more exclusively on the parasite. It consists in having the patient go at least 24 hours with nothing to eat but liquid foods, and even these in rather limited amounts. At the same time mild laxatives, as castor oil, may be employed to still further empty the bowel. Shortly before taking the medicine it is a good idea to have the patient take a moderate portion of smoked herring, onion or garlic. These foods seem distasteful to the worm and assist in its expulsion. The most reliable medicine to give is filix mas, or as it is more commonly called, male fern. A good way to give it is as follows:—

℞.—Oleoresin filicis macis   2 drams.

Sig.—Put into nine capsules. Take three capsules every two hours. In two hours after taking the last dose, take two ounces of castor oil.

Many other remedies besides male fern have been used, such as emulsion of pumpkin seeds; blossoms of kousso, 5 to 8 drams in infusion; decoction of pomegranate root, 2 ounces; pelletierin tannate, 5 to 15 grains; kamala, 3 to 4 drams; cocoanut milk; salol; benzin; naphthalin and many others, but none of them are better than the male fern, and that offers the advantages of being fairly easy to take when put into capsules, and is also cheap.

Of the nematodes, the only ones of interest to us in this country, are ascaris lumbricoides, the oxyuris vermiformis, the trichina spiralis and the uncinaria duodenalis.

The ascaris lumbricoides, or long round worm, is very frequently found in the human intestine. It is brown, red or yellow in color, cylindrical in shape, and looks like the common earth worm. The size varies, the male being from twenty to twenty-five centimeters long, the female from thirty to forty. The head has three cone-shaped lips, and fine teeth, numbering about 200. There are four longitudinal lines running from head to tail, and numerous cross striations. At the tail end of the male is a cloaca from which project several spiculæ, these being the copulative organs. From the junction of the first and second thirds, on the abdominal lines of the female, is the sexual opening, and entering into it, two long stretched uteri. Their fecundity is something enormous, the number of eggs in a pregnant female being estimated at 60,000,000. These ˗ ˗ ˞s are small, dark and oval. The parasite is found in the small intestine. Unlike the tænia, they require no host, but gain access to the body in the form of embryos which are present in vegetables, fruit, and water, or may be transmitted from one person directly to another.

Symptomatology:—Symptoms may be absent, or if present they may be obscure and consist of various digestive or nervous symptoms, with nothing distinctive about them. Increased appetite, anorexia, belching and sometimes more or less pain may be present.

Diagnosis:—This can be made only by finding the parasite or some of its eggs in the fæcal passages.

Treatment:—Preventive treatment consists in careful cleansing or thorough cooking of foods, and care that drinking water be not infected. Because of lack of attention to these details, these parasites are more common in the uncivilized, the insane and in children. For the purpose of expelling the ascarides, santonin may be used. This may be given as the crude drug, $\frac{1}{4}$ to 1 grain three times a day, or it may be given in the attenuation. A good way is to give santonin 1x or 2x, one or two tablets before each meal. A combination frequently used is santonin $\frac{1}{4}$ grain, and calomel 1 to 2 grains. This acts as a laxative as well as a vermifuge, and so helps to expel the parasites as well as to destroy them.

The oxyuris vermiformis, or pin worm, is a small, white, thread-like worm. The male is about five, the female, about twelve millimeters long. The head of each is a small knob, the mouth has three lips, the tail is blunt. At first the parasite is in the small intestine, later it passes to the large, thence the female passes to the rectum and is expelled. The eggs are not liberated until it has left the body; then, if they get into food or drinking water, or are on the fingers of a child, they may get into the mouth of an individual, who thus becomes infected.

Symptomatology:—When in the small intestine, pin worms cause no symptoms of themselves, but by their irritation of the mucosa, enteritis may develop, causing diarrhœa. When present about the rectum and anus, a severe itching is produced. This is generally the most prominent symptom. It is especially manifest in the lower bowel, but may extend to the outside, and in little girls often extends to the vagina and vulva.

Diagnosis:—This can be made with certainty only by finding the parasites in the stool. The laity have an idea that restlessness in sleep, chewing movements, picking of the nose, and fever, especially at night, are caused by worms. Undoubtedly this may be true at times, but a diagnosis can certainly not be made upon such symptoms, as they may be caused by too hearty eating, indigestion and other conditions.

Treatment:—Santonin, the same as for the ascaris lumbricoides, is useful although it does not seem to be as uniformly successful as for that parasite. Spigelia is also a remedy that often proves useful, given in the 2x or 3x. In addition to the remedy, it is well to wash the rectum out with one quart of water to which four tablespoonfuls of salt have been added, or ½ tablespoonful of vinegar. If excessive itching is present, it may indicate that a mass of the worms is lying in the rectum. A gocd enæma to remove them is thymol, 1 part to 100 parts of olive oil. The mild mercurial ointment may also be smeared about the anus to relieve itching. Treatment for these worms should be kept up for sometime, until careful examination of the stool fails to reveal their presence. Usually this will take two or three weeks at least.

Infection by the trichina spiralis is caused by eating pork containing the parasites. There are three stages of the disease:—

1.—The intestinal stage. The symptoms arising from their presence in the intestine usually appear in a day or two after eating food containing the trichinae and consist of anorexia, nausea, vomiting, diarrhœa and colicky pain.

2.—The migratory stage, in which the parasite penetrates through the wall of the intestine and migrates to any of the muscles of the body. During this stage there is severe pain in the muscles, simulating very closely the pain of muscular rheumatism. There is also fever, prostration, nausea, stiffness of the muscles, some swelling or œdema, insomnia and frequently delirium.

3.—The stage of encapsulation. Death may take place during either of the first two stages, but if it does not, after two or three weeks the inflammatory process existing around the parasite results in the formation of a capsule which encloses it. Under the microscope it then appears coiled up in the enclosure. It is large enough so that the muscle containing a number of them appears granular to the naked eye.

Diagnosis:—Trichina spiralis may be suspected if the above symptoms come on after eating pork, but can be proven to exist only by finding them in the fæces, or in a small portion of excised muscle. Of the skeletal muscles, they are most frequently found in the deltoid.

Prognosis:—This depends largely upon the number of parasites taken into the system, and also upon the strength and resisting power of the individual. Patients sometimes die from the severity of the gastro-intestinal symptoms, but more frequently death occurs after the parasites have reached the muscles and organs of the body. However, quite a proportion of cases recover after a more or less prolonged sickness, and regain comparatively good health.

Treatment:—Prophylaxis consists in thorough meat inspection, or thorough cooking. If infection has occurred, and is diagnosed soon, washing out of the stomach and colon will be beneficial, thus removing as many of the parasites as possible before they are absorbed. Some remedy should then be given in an effort to destroy those still remaining in the stomach or intestine. For this purpose, nothing is better than salol, 5 grain doses three or four times a day. Glycerine given freely is also beneficial. After muscular symptoms arise, they should be treated the same as if due to rheumatism, which they so closely resemble. For this purpose, rest, hot applications and the indicated remedy may be employed.

The uncinaria duodenale or hook-worm has been known for centuries, and is said to have been mentioned by Egyptian writers of three and four thousand years ago. In the tropics of Asia and Africa, and in the islands of the lower latitudes, the parasites have caused great ravages ever since. Until recent years they were thought to be rare in this country except in emigrants from foreign parts. In 1902 Stiles reported the frequent finding of a parasite of similar shape and habits in the southern states. At first his findings were discredited, but ultimately they have been found to be correct, and much importance is now attached to the effects produced by this parasite upon the health of the southern people.

In this country, the technical name of uncinaria Americana, or common name of hookworm has been given to the parasite. The length of the male is about 10 to 11 mm., of the female 18 mm. They have several sharp teeth with which a firm hold is taken upon the mucous membrane of the intestine. Leading from the mouth is a muscular œsophagus, by means of which blood is sucked from its host. The eggs are oval in shape and given off in great numbers. It has been claimed that the number of ova found in the stool indicates the number of parasites; 150 to 180 ova to the cubic centimeter of fæces indicate 1,000 worms. They are found chiefly in the jejunum, but to some extent in the duodenum and sometimes in the colon. They need no intermediate host. The ova gaining access to drinking water, food, or the dirt upon the hands or under the finger nails are carried to the mouth and then pass into the stomach and intestine. It is also claimed that they may penetrate the skin, for instance in people who go barefoot. They are then carried by the blood to the heart, thence into the pulmonary circulation, whence the embryonic parasites penetrate the lung tissue into the bronchial tubes, and being coughed into the pharynx, pass into the stomach and intestine.

The symptoms are chiefly due to their sucking the blood from their host, thus causing anæmia. Three stages are mentioned. In the first, there are signs of intestinal irritation, with possibly some fever. In the second, there is pronounced anæmia, resembling the progressive pernicious form, and accompanied with much languor and prostration. The skin is of a muddy hue, the eyes are dull and lack expression. If children reach this stage, their growth is stunted and they become ill developed. In the third stage, the liver and spleen become enlarged, the intestinal walls are thickened, effusion takes place into the abdomen and the feet become œdematous.

Diagnosis :—This is made by finding the ova or parasites in the stools.

Treatment :—Prophylaxis should include sanitary care of fæces from infected individuals. Attention should be given to the drinking water; food should be carefully washed or cooked; there should be cleanliness of the person so that they may not accumulate on the surface of the body and penetrate the skin, and shoes with good soles should be worn for the same purpose.

In the curative treatment of those infected, thymol has given the best results. The patient should be prepared by a few days of light diet. One-half dram of thymol is then given, the same dose to be repeated in two hours. After another two hours, a dose of castor oil is used. This treatment often needs to be given several times in order to remove all the parasites and ova, and then extra care should be taken that the patient is not re-infected. Male fern given in the same manner as for tape-worms is also a successful treatment.

The trematodes or fluke-like worms are but seldom seen in this country, and when they are found are always in people who have lived in Asiatic countries. There are several varieties, but owing to their rarity they will not be discussed here, except to say that their symptoms, diagnosis and treatment are all practically the same as for the other varieties of parasites.

CHAPTER XVI.

INTESTINAL AUTO-INTOXICATION.

Opinions differ widely in regard to the importance of this condition. Some consider it to be of such slight consequence that the symptoms arising from it are given little attention. Others, especially those who have taken up with the writings of Bouchard, and more recently those of Metchnikoff, believe that the poisons generated in the intestine and absorbed into the blood have a great influence upon the health of the individual. Probably the truth of the matter lies about midway between these two extremes.

That disturbances, not only of the digestive processes but also of the functions of other organs and of the general health, are sometimes present as a result of intestinal toxins, is undoubtedly true. But that the widespread and serious affections sometimes attributed to them are really caused by these toxins, can hardly be believed.

In the broadest sense injurious agents arising from the intestinal contents are of two kinds:—

1.—Bacteria.

2.—The products of bacteria.

Under certain pathological conditions various bacteria may be absorbed by the blood vessels or lymphatics of the intestine, carried to other localities, and there produce suppurative or other diseased states. The bacillus coli communis is especially prone to act in this way. Troubles caused by the bacteria themselves however, are generally of a surgical nature, and therefore will not be considered at this time.

Auto-intoxication in a medical sense is caused by poisonous materials resulting from the action of bacteria upon the food contained in the intestine. Very little is absolutely known in regard to the nature of the toxic substances. Different chemical agents and compounds have been mentioned, some of which are undoubtedly active as poisons; no doubt many others of which chemistry is ignorant at this time are also injurious. Ptomaines and leucomaines are the general names given to those which are supposed to act most viciously upon the health. As indicated by their names, they are chiefly derived from nitrogenous substances, although quite likely some inorganic substances and also some derived from other than nitrogenous sources are capable of acting deleteriously. However, the whole matter is so imperfectly understood, and is so largely theoretical that it has no place in this article. The same is true as regards the varieties of bacteria through whose activities the toxins are formed, although it may be said that those which produce putrefaction are the ones supposed to be chiefly responsible. It is not thought that any special or unusual forms are necessary, but that those normally present in the intestine act in producing these toxins when certain conditions exist.

Etiology :—For the development of the materials which cause auto-intoxication, and for the induction of the symptoms themselves, two factors seem of importance. These are,—

1.—Stagnation of the bowel contents.

2.—An irritated state of the mucous lining.

Bacteria multiply more rapidly in any reservoir or channel from which there is sluggish drainage. The intestinal canal is no exception to this rule. Therefore if in an individual there is either constipation or obstipation the intestinal bacteria will be more numerous and their effects more pronounced. Because of the greater tendency to formation and absorption of the toxic principles where the intestinal current is slow, it is probable that in most cases the symptoms of auto-intoxication are caused by processes taking place in the large bowel; although if an ileus takes place, and possibly to some extent at other times, these poisons may be formed in the small intestine. Metchnikoff has given emphasis to the idea that putrefactive changes taking place in the colon have a great influence in affecting the entire organism, even to the extent of inducing sclerotic changes of the blood vessels and other organs of the body; also, that the pathological conditions associated with old age are hastened to a great extent by colonic putrefaction.

An irritated state of the mucous membrane lining the colon, such as a chronic enteritis, or even a chronic congestion, seems to help materially in producing auto-intoxication, obtaining from three different sources.

1.—The effects of a congested or thickened condition of the mucous membrane is likely to extend somewhat to the musculature of the intestinal wall, and thus weaken peristalsis.

2.—A catarrhal or congested state of the mucous membrane is a fertile field for bacterial growth.

3.—Such a membranous lining seems to offer less resistance to toxic materials in gaining access to the blood stream.

Anything of a nature irritating to the lining of the bowel therefore predisposes to auto-intoxication. Undoubtedly the bacteria and their products themselves, have an effect in this direction. The same may be said of the physical pressure of hardened fæces. Lastly, no doubt, many of the popular laxatives and cathartics, although they temporarily relieve constipation, are injurious because of their irritating effects.

Symptomatology:—The symptoms of intestinal auto-intoxication may be considered from two standpoints:

1.—Those manifested by the intestinal tract itself.

2.—Those which are produced by the action of the absorbed toxins upon other organs.

Of the digestive symptoms present, it is difficult to decide to what extent they are dependent upon the toxins. They are chiefly of a nature which might be expected to arise from constipation alone. They may be due to some primary digestive abnormality, which produces constipation, and is thus indirectly causative of the intoxication instead of its symptom. Whether understood as cause or effect it may be said that there is generally anorexia, coated tongue, bad taste, flatulence and sometimes more or less abdominal pain and tenderness.

Other organs which are most apt to be affected in this trouble are:—

1.—The skin.
2.—The kidneys.
3.—The respiratory system.
4.—The lymphatics.
5.—The circulatory system.
6.—The nervous system.

The skin being an eliminative organ is evidently called upon to remove from the system some of the toxins which have been absorbed into the blood. In performing this act, more or less injury is done to the skin itself and the excretory glands contained in it. There is apt to be an abnormal dryness, a pale or muddy color and there may be several types of skin diseases with their eruptions and other symptoms.

The kidneys are also irritated in their efforts to eliminate the poisonous materials. No doubt cirrhosis of these organs is sometimes caused, or at least the process is hastened as a result of the damage done in this manner. An examination of the urine is of especial interest because of the fact that in auto-intoxication, indican is so often found. The importance of its detection is a matter of some uncertainty. There are writers who emphasize it to the extent of declaring that its presence is necessary in a genuine case of this trouble, and who determine the success of their treatment upon its effect in removing it from the urine. There are others who although admitting its relationship to an undue putrefaction in the intestinal tract, yet do not consider its presence or its absence of such decisive importance. Undoubtedly, taken together with other signs, it is of considerable value.

The air cells and mucous membrane of the respiratory tract may share in the irritation caused by efforts in oxygenating these toxic products. As a result bronchitis and catarrhal processes are frequently present.

The lymphatics are almost as active in absorbing intestinal toxins as are the blood vessels. As a result, the lymphatic glands may suffer injury. It is difficult to determine of how much consequence this is in the development of scrofula and other diseased conditions of these glands. It can be said, however, that removing the conditions giving rise to auto-intoxication is of material benefit in the treatment of diseases of the lymphatics.

The circulatory system, in transporting the poisons to the various eliminative organs, suffers from damage done in transit. Arterio-sclerosis is undoubtedly hastened by the injuries done to the vessel walls in this manner. The heart is also damaged by the passage of the toxic matters through its caliber as well as by the blood circulating in its walls for its own nutrition. In addition to these direct effects upon the circulatory system, its functions are modified to a considerable extent by the influence of the poisons upon the vaso motor and other nerve centers controlling the circulation of the blood.

The symptoms and lesions so far mentioned are due largely to the irritating properties of the offending materials. Like other alkaloidal poisons, however, the real toxic effects from a physiological standpoint are chiefly exerted upon the nervous system. The milder symptoms are drowsiness, insomnia, irritability, melancholia and neuralgia. The patient feels drowsy and inactive, yet when sleep is attemtped it is unsatisfactory. Insomnia due either to a restless feeling or to mental anxiety is apt to be present, or if sleep is attained it is fitful and accompanied with unpleasant dreams. There is apt to be an undue irritability of temper which makes life unpleasant to the sufferer and also to his associates. This tendency instead of manifesting itself as an excitability of temper may be in the form of a moroseness and menlancholia.

Functional diseases of the nervous system such as neurasthenia and hysteria are common with intestinal auto-intoxication. Some have expressed the opinion that these diseases are but symptoms of the condition under consideration. To some extent, this may be true; on the other hand it seems just as reasonable to believe that neurasthenia, for instance, is an evidence of a nervous stigma, just the same as auto-intoxication is the result of an imperfectly developed or functioning digestive system. It seems quite likely that both of these conditions are in this way evidences of the same primary tendencies of the individual's personality. Epilepsy is sometimes associated with evidences of auto-intoxication, and cases have been reported that were materially benefited by correcting the intestinal conditions. Certain forms of functional insanity are also said to be induced or at least aggravated by putrefactive products absorbed from the bowel. In all these nervous and mental troubles, it seems best to consider that abnormal or morbid tendencies must first have existed. Then, if intestinal toxins are absorbed, they act as exciting causes, and the fully developed affections arise.

Diagnosis:—Where either functional or organic diseases of the digestive tract are present, associated with flatulence, usually with constipation, restless sleep, vertigo and dry and unhealthy skin, one should suspect intestinal putrefaction and auto-intoxication. If the urine contains evidences of putrefactive products, especially indican, the diagnosis may be safely assumed. In considering this trouble, one should recognize its possible influence in materially impairing the health, yet the mistake should not be made of attaching undue importance to it. Many times it is dependent upon or associated with some other affection of equal or superior importance.

Treatment:—Being so frequently a concomitant of some other disease, successful treatment is often dependent upon remedying the associated condition as for instance, the digestive trouble which gives rise to constipation. The gastroptosis, displaced uterus, hypertrophied rectal valves, adherent appendix, or other abdominal difficulties which interfere with intestinal evacuations may all have to be treated medically or surgically. Constitutional diseases which depress or modify gastro-intestinal activities may need to be remedied. Treatment of the condition itself may be considered from three standpoints:

1.—Preventing so far as possible the formation of the poisonous agents.

2.—Removal from the body of the toxins that are formed.

3.—Treating the results produced by the poisons upon the body.

In preventing the formation of the toxic agents, attention should be given to the diet from which they are derived, and to the bacteria which are active in their production. These toxins are thought to be developed chiefly
by putrefactive processes taking place upon nitrogenous
foods. For this reason it is often advisable to reduce somewhat the amount which is being eaten of this class of
foods, being sure not to allow more than can be well digested. What this amount should be may often be determined to a considerable extent by the manner in which
the secretory and motor functions of the stomach and intestine are performed. For instance, if secretion of the
gastric ferments is deficient, foods of an albuminous nature will enter the intestine in an imperfectly prepared
condition, and therefore will be more susceptible to the
action of putrefactive bacteria because of this fact. In
the same way, if others of the abnormal conditions described in previous chapters are present, the diet selected
in accordance with the suggestions in those chapters will
ordinarily be the best one in a case suffering from auto-
intoxication. Some have advised that these cases be put
upon an exclusive milk diet for a time. This may give
good results in those individuals who can satisfactorily
digest casein and cream, but there are those who will do
but poorly upon this diet. A vegetable diet has also been
recommended with the idea that it does not contain as
much putrefactive material as do the meats, but it often
fails. Some of the most difficult cases of indigestion and
auto-intoxication which one is called upon to treat, are
amongst vegetarians. Getting along upon a low diet, so as
to limit the amount of putrefactive material in the intestine, may be useful for a time, but it is sometimes carried
too far and kept up too long, and then the neurasthenic

and other symptoms which are to some extent dependent upon a poor state of nutrition will be aggravated, and the digestive powers will be still further disabled. It seems, therefore, as in the treatment of all digestive troubles, it is best not to go to extremes, or to follow some dietetic fad, but to select a diet which is as agreeable as possible to the patient's taste, which is sufficient to produce a good state of nutrition without being excessive, which meets as far as can be determined the functional capacities of the digestive functions, which is well prepared and is fresh. Taking food which is already beginning to undergo putrefaction, as so-called seasoned meat, may cause or aggravate the trouble.

For the purpose of limiting the number of intestinal bacteria and their activities, not very much can be done except to overcome the constipation, and this will be considered later. So-called intestinal antiseptics have been much employed in late years for the purpose of destroying the bacteria or at least inhibiting their activities. Success in their use has not been very great, however. This may be accounted for by the fact that antiseptic or other agents are so changed in their passage through the stomach and the small intestine that by the time the large intestine is reached, where they are chiefly needed, they are not of much utility. Another reason why these substances are not of very much service in the trouble under consideration, is that they are more or less irritating to the mucous membrane and so give rise to one of the factors involved in causing auto-intoxication. As the value of these agents is so limited, and as attention to the diet and overcoming the constipation is of so much more consequence in decreasing the number of bacteria, no further attention will be given to their consideration.

In removing the toxic products from the body, the treatment outlined in the chapter on constipation is applicable, except in the rare cases which already have sufficiently free bowel movements, and are seemingly entirely dependent upon the second of the etiological factors; that is, an irritated state of the mucous lining. A suitable diet for the constipation should be selected so far as practicable, and other general methods such as exercises, massage, vibration, hydrotherapy and electricity may all be employed, so long as one does not go to extremes and give some of them undue importance in this connection. Enemata may often be employed advantageously for a time. Best results will be obtained by the patient's assuming the knee chest position and allowing the fluid to enter the rectum and colon rather slowly from a fountain syringe. Plain warm water, a salt solution or soap and water may be employed, an effort being made to retain the enema for a few minutes, until it gravitates as far as possible into the bowel. This treatment carried out every night for a time will often make the patient feel brighter, stronger and better in every way. It has its drawback, however, if continued very long, for it seems to accustom the bowel to the presence of foreign matter, and the bowel still further loses its inclination to expel the fæces. If diet and physical methods do not suffice to overcome the constipation sufficiently, resort may be had to the remedies mentioned under constipation. If absolutely necessary, the laxatives there mentioned may also be employed. If these latter are used, care should be exercised to select only those which are as little irritating to the mucous membrane as possible. The salines are quite useful for producing a quick and free evacuation, thus removing the toxins and many of the bacteria, but if frequently used they have a very decidedly irritating effect. Some of the vegetable drugs are also of that nature, as jalap, elaterium, and to some extent aloin. Any of these or castor oil may be used temporarily, where an immediate effect is desired, but should not be continued for any length of time. Some agent to develop the strength of the intestinal musculature seems most desirable. For this purpose cascara sagrada gives excellent results. In intestinal auto-intoxication a compound composed of two parts fluid extract cascara sagrada, and one part each of glycerine and simple aromatic elixir, is very satisfactory for continued use. The glycerine seems to have some inhibiting effect upon putrefactive activities. Of this preparation one teaspoonful may be given after each meal. Often this dose may be gradually diminished, as the constipation and other symptoms improve, until finally it may be possible to stop it altogether and get along without a laxative. Phenolthallein is another agent which has come into quite frequent use recently in cases of the kind. Given in one to three grain doses at night, it often does excellent service, and has the advantages of being agreeable to take, and causing no griping.

Attention should also be given to promoting the elimination of those toxins which have been absorbed into the blood current or by the lymphatics. This may be done by such means as keeping the skin clean and hygienic by the free use of hydrotherapeutic methods. The living and sleeping rooms should be well ventilated so that irritating substances seeking exit from the body by way of the respiratory tract may be promptly oxygenated. Water should be freely imbibed for the purpose of keeping the kidneys thoroughly flushed, that the injurious substances passing out of the system in this direction may be as rapidly and completely excreted as possible. Plenty of outdoor exercise and other means of improving the circulation and metabolism of the body should be employed, for by so doing it seems that even when toxic products have been absorbed from the intestine they may yet to some extent be changed into inert or nutritive substances by means of the metabolic capabilities of the liver, muscles and other tissues and organs of the body.

Treating the results produced upon the body by the poisons is too extensive a subject to take up in this chapter. In fact it may be more appropriately considered under the various diseased conditions which are produced in this manner, for instance, in the consideration of diseases of the skin, the kidneys, the circulatory system and the nervous and mental conditions in which auto-intoxication is of etiological importance. Perhaps it would be more closely associated with the purpose of this volume to consider the remedies which may have an influence in this trouble in its digestive manifestations, but these have been sufficiently noticed in the chapters describing these various affections.

Part IV.—Diseases of the Bile Tract.

CHAPTER I.

JAUNDICE OR ICTERUS.

Definition:—A condition where the skin, mucous membranes and fluids of the body are yellowish in color, as a result of bile pigment in the blood. The intensity of the yellowish color may vary from such a slight tinge that it is hardly distinguishable, to one so dark that it is sometimes called black jaundice. It usually first appears in the conjunctivae, and may be confined to these membranes. It is but a symptom, and may be found in various diseases, but from its importance it seems well to give it some consideration.

Etiology:—In whatever disease it may be found it is a result of one or the other of two conditions:

1.—Obstruction in some part of the bile ducts.

2.—Some form of toxæmia.

In the obstructive form, the interference is with the free passage of the bile into the intestine; it is blocked back into the branches of the bile duct in the liver, is absorbed into the radicles of the hepatic vein, and in this way reaches the general circulation. The obstruction may be due to a catarrhal process in the duct or at its entrance into the duodenum, to the lodgment in it of a gall stone, to cicatricial tissue, to pancreatic disease at the point where the common duct passes through its head, or to pressure by a tumor located in some adjacent organ as the stomach, kidney, omentum, pancreas or liver.

215

In the toxæmic form there is circulating in the blood some poison which causes disintegration of the red corpuscles, with liberation of hæmoglobin, this resulting in an increased formation of bile pigments. Toxæmic jaundice may be found in a variety of the infectious diseases, such as malaria, typhoid, scarlet and yellow fever, pneumonia and pyæmia. Certain of the chemical poisons may also produce it, such as phosphorus, mercury, arsenic, antimony, copper and snake venom.

Symptomatology:—This varies considerably, depending upon the cause, the severity and the duration of the attack. If severe and long lasting the skin is apt not only to be yellowish in color, but may develop a pruritus. Undue sweating, urticaria, and boils may also be present. Of the secretions, the urine is especially apt to be colored, and frequently, also, the tears, saliva and milk. Where obstruction prevents bile from entering the intestine the stools become clay-colored; this is partly due to the absence of bile, and partly results from the presence of undigested fat. In the toxæmic form the stools may be unduly colored with bile. Especially in the early stages of jaundice, the pulse and respirations are apt to be lessened in frequency. There is an increased tendency to hæmorrhage, and in case of an injury, or if an operation becomes necessary, this tendency to bleed may be extremely difficult to control. At other times it may manifest itself in the form of a purpura, or subcutaneous hæmorrhage. Mental symptoms sometimes develop, there being irritability, melancholia, and in severe protracted cases, coma, delirium and convulsions.

The treatment depends upon the disease or condition giving rise to the jaundice, and therefore should be considered under those heads.

CHAPTER II.

CHOLANGITIS.

Definition:—An inflammatory process in the bile ducts, may manifest itself in any one of the following conditions:
1.—Catarrhal cholangitis.
2.—Croupous cholangitis.
3.—Suppurative cholangitis.
4.—Ulcerative cholangitis.

CATARRHAL CHOLANGITIS.

Definition:—A catarrhal inflammation affecting the bile ducts, may be either acute or chronic. The acute form has the following:

Etiology:—In the vast majority of cases it is an extension of the same condition affecting the duodenum. Eating food in excessive quantities, or an injudicious selection of food is apt to give rise to both the duodenitis and the cholangitis. It may also be caused by an extension from other sources, such as from the substance of the liver, the pancreas, and possibly from the lungs. It may be caused by injury,—as by the passage of gall stones. It is also an accompaniment of certain of the infectious diseases, notably malaria, typhoid and cholera. The importance of bacteria in the causation of diseases of the bile tract has been considerably dwelt upon in recent years and undoubtedly in many cases they play an important part. In fact strictly speaking it is probable that bacteria of some sort assist in the etiology of all cases.

Symptomatology:—As it is most frequently a sequel to gastro-enteritis, the symptoms of this condition are of course present. Some of these symptoms are increased in severity by the cholangitis, and some new symptoms are added. That is, the prostration, vertigo, and possibly

fever which were present with the duodenitis are increased. Of the additional symptoms icterus is the most
characteristic; this appears in a few days, and is variable
in degree and persistency, depending upon the severity of
the process. In addition to being jaundiced, the skin frequently itches a great deal. In many cases an urticaria
develops. The urine becomes yellow from the presence of
biliary acids, and the stools become light colored from the
decrease of the acids in the bowels. The jaundice, yellow
urine and light colored stools result from the swelling of
the lining of the ducts interfering with the free passage
of the bile into the intestine; but as the swelling is not apt
to be so severe as to cause complete obstruction to the
passage of the bile, the jaundice is not often as marked
as when a gall stone completely occludes the duct. As
some bile generally passes to the bowel, the stools are not
of that clay color that is associated with gall stone. Sometimes there is tenderness and even pain in the region of
the liver, although these features are not present unless
the liver becomes congested and enlarged; conditions which
are comparatively rare in cholangitis alone, being present
probably only where the bacterial infection is especially
pronounced.

The duration of acute cholangitis is variable. Sometimes it is only transient, or is a so-called abortive attack.
At other times it persists until it must be classed as chronic,—a description of which follows. However in the majority of cases it lasts two or three weeks, and then gradually disappears. Convalescence, even after it is commenced, is often quite prolonged, considerably more so
than in ordinary acute gastro-enteritis. Cases are sometimes seen which considerably resemble typhoid fever; in
fact it occasionally seems appropriate to make a diagnosis

of typhoid with cholangitis complications. At such times of course the symptoms, especially the fever and prostration are more severe, and usually longer lasting. Such severe attacks have by some writers been described as a separate entity under the name of Weil's disease, and it has been claimed that as regards cause, it is very closely related to typhoid, but so far no proof has been found to this effect. Sequelæ which may develop are chronic cholangitis, suppurative cholangitis and cholecystitis.

Pathology:—Opportunities for post-mortem work on uncomplicated cases of acute catarrhal cholangitis are rare. It is presumed however that the ordinary changes found in acute inflammations of the mucous membrane elsewhere, are present, such as excessive secretions of mucus, loosening of epithelium and an accumulation of leucocytes. The presence of this compound of mucus, leucocytes and epithelium, together with the swelling of the membrane, causes partial obstruction of the ducts, blocking to some extent the flow of bile, thus allowing its absorption into the blood, with the resulting jaundice. Nothing very definite is known as to the portion of the ducts most severely involved, but it is probably sometimes the lower and larger ducts, and sometimes the smaller ramifications penetrating the liver.

Diagnosis:—When associated with an acute gastro-enteritis, with the ordinary causes of such condition, the diagnosis is easy, although its origin is sometimes obscure. For instance a gall stone may pass without causing the characteristic pain, but producing a traumatic cholangitis. A neoplasm of some surrounding part may also suddenly reach such a size or position as to set up the condition by pressure. In a few cases as mentioned in the symptomatology, attacks will occur closely resembling typhoid fever.

In these conditions a close study is necessary, looking for the various symptoms of these affections, and diagnosing by exclusion.

Chronic catarrhal cholangitis is frequently a sequel to an acute attack. At other times it is a result of some continuously acting cause, such as extension of a chronic inflammation from the parenchyma of the liver, which inflammation may be due to cancer, hydatids or other long lasting conditions of the liver. The irritation produced by the pressure of a gall stone is a frequent cause, but probably the one most often acting is the migration of bacteria from the duodenum up the common duct.

Symptomatology :—The chief symptom of simple chronic catarrhal cholangitis is the icterus. This may not be as marked as in an acute attack, or it may present frequent exacerbations, depending upon the variations in the intensity of the pathology present. These exacerbations may be accompanied by the same constitutional symptoms which go with the acute form. When the trouble is associated with gall stones these periodical aggravations are apt to be more marked. Bits or plugs of mucus sometimes form, hard enough so that in passing they may cause such severe pains as to be mistaken for the passing of a gall stone. In considering cholelithiasis it will be remarked that such bits of mucus, more likely those in the gall bladder, but sometimes those in the ducts, often form the nucleus to which cholesterin crystals adhere, thus giving rise to the concretions.

CROUPOUS CHOLANGITIS.

A very few cases have been reported where the mucous membranes lining the bile ducts have been covered by a croupous membrane; these have sometimes passed away as casts. When this occurs, severe pain, simulating true gall stone colic is present. In fact operations have been performed with the expectation of finding gall stones,— yet upon reaching the gall bladder and ducts, no stones were found, though there would be evidences of a false membrane,—croupous or diphtheritic in nature, involving both the ducts and the bladder. The symptoms are icterus, and pain as of hepatic colic.

SUPPURATIVE CHOLANGITIS.

Etiology:—This form is always due to bacterial infection. It has been considered in the past that bile possesses an antiseptic action. If this were true, it would not be expected that bacteria could develop in the biliary ducts, —constantly bathed as they are in the bile. In recent years however, experiment has shown that the antiseptic action of bile is very limited. It has been demonstrated that when the liver and ducts are in a healthy condition, the bile is at least sterile, but when these organs become diseased, bacteria may gain entrance and multiply. The pathway by which infection usually enters, is undoubtedly through the orifice from the intestine. It passes upward in opposition to the bile current, and may reach the finest ramifications of the ducts. It naturally travels thus against the bile current in people who from anatomical conformity, lack of exercise, or for some other reason possess a stagnation, or reduced velocity of bile movement. Two other occasional methods may be mentioned by which bacteria may gain access to the bile; they may penetrate the walls of the gall bladder directly from some other organ, or they may be carried there by the blood current.

The form of bacteria most commonly found in this condition, is the bacillus coli communis. This is found in all persons the entire length of the intestinal canal. In health it is not pathogenic, but in morbid states it may produce any one of several conditions. In this case it will be a suppurative cholangitis. The streptococci and the staphylococci may act as causative agents. Sometimes they exist in connection with the B. coli communis, at other times they may be alone. The bacteria of typhoid, cholera and pneumonia may also act etiologically.

Investigation has revealed the fact that the various bacteria above mentioned are often present in the bile passages without giving rise to suppuration. At other times they will produce it to an extreme degree. Just the cause of this is difficult to determine, but it is probably a difference either in the virulence of the bacteria, or in the resisting power of the tissues. For instance, if the tissues have been bruised or injured by the passage of gall stones, or other injury, a temporary traumatic inflammation may develop; then if any form of bacteria gain access, they act like a torch to inflammable material.

Pathology :—The secretion in suppurative cholangitis contains numerous cells, and resembles pus,—rather than the mucus which is found in the catarrhal form. In the earlier stages there is a small-celled infiltration of the walls of the bile passages and their surroundings, which if long continued develops into a connective tissue thickening. Usually owing to this thickening there is obstruction to the outflow of both the bile and the pus. As a result, dilatations will be produced,—a condition resembling bronchiectasis such as occurs in the lungs. If the finer bile passages permeating the liver are involved, very small accumulations of pus appear in the lobules. These frequently develop into abscesses, and result in disintegration of the liver substance. A number of these small abscesses may unite, forming one large abscess which may involve a large area.

Symptomatology :—The symptoms vary somewhat, depending upon the kind of infection, also upon whether there is any other existing disease or complication, that is, whether there is an associated cholelithiasis, typhoid, cholera, or pneumonia. In these latter conditions however the pus is not apt to form until convalescence is establishe l. Cases have been reported where weeks, months or even years after having recovered from typhoid, the patient had developed a suppurative chcolangitis, which upon investigation would present typhoid bacilli in the secretions. At other times these bacilli have been found in the bile passages as long as seven years after an attack of the fever, without suppuration having developed. Icterus as a symptom is not as marked as in the catarrhal variety. When present to any extent it is usually due to some occlusion which may have existed before the suppuration, and not to the suppuration itself. Fever is often present, and it is then one of the most important symptoms. As usual when fever is due to suppurative processes, it is either remitting or intermitting. It is often low or absent in the morning, and high at night. For this reason it has often been mistaken for malaria,—also sometimes for tuberculosis. In other cases it will be very irregular. Sometimes there is chill, followed by fever, with sweat during its defervescence. There is also frequently an enlargement of the spleen, and as a result of this the trouble may be mistaken for typhoid. Poisons producing noxious effects on the kidneys, heart or other organs are sometimes developed. Pain or tenderness over the region of the liver is often present. If the gall bladder is involved, as it frequently is, the pain is apt to be severe.

Diagnosis:—If there has been a history of gall stones, or trouble with the bile passages, followed by some disease in which infectious germs are present either in the intestine or blood,—or if the B. coli communis is present without such preceding disease, and there should arise an irregular fever, with pain and tenderness in this region, icterus slight or absent, and an enlarged spleen, one is justified in looking for suppurative cholangitis, or cholecystitis. It may be differentiated from malaria by the absence of the plasmodium, from typhoid by the absence of the rose spots and the Widal reaction, from tuberculosis by the absence of pulmonary signs and the bacilli. It may be impossible to differentiate from abscess of the liver without bile duct complication, but this may sometimes be done by the greater pain in that trouble, its history, the usual entire absence of icterus and the physical signs which go with that disease.

Prognosis:—In most cases it is grave. If as often happens there is obstruction by cholelithic or other agent, there are dangers both from stoppage of the bile, and from the pus being blocked back into the liver causing multiple abscesses in that organ. However if spontaneous or operative removal of the obstruction can be effected, followed by thorough drainage, recovery may ensue.

ULCERATIVE CHOLANGITIS.

This may be an accompaniment of some of the other forms, especially the suppurative. It is usually due to pressure by a gall stone or other concretion on a circumscribed spot of the bile duct. Cancer, tuberculosis, typhoid and cholera, are also said to have acted as causes.

The point of chief importance in regard to it, is to remember that the ulceration may result in perforation of the wall, causing of course acute peritonitis. A stricture or fistula may be produced, or hæmorrhage may result, or the ulcerative process may penetrate just deep enough to cause a plastic inflammation of the serous covering, resulting in localized adhesions. This may be considered salutary in a way, because it prevents perforation with general peritonitis, yet the anchoring by adhesions of these organs, the liver, gall bladder, ducts, stomach, duodenum and jejunum, often causes obscure digestive troubles. Many such cases have been treated for years as indigestion, gastritis or neuroses, when in reality the pylorus, duodenum or some part was so bound to some other part as a result of adhesions resulting from cholangitis, that peristalsis could not be properly performed until the adhesions were liberated, and resulting from such interference the digestive symptoms were present.

CHAPTER III.

CHOLECYSTITIS.

Inflammation of the gall bladder is very closely associated, as a rule, with the same pathological condition of the ducts; and in a vast majority of cases it is simply an extension of the inflammation. Possibly in exceptional cases the causative agent may gain access directly through the walls of the gall bladder itself, but the usual course is by entering the common duct from the duodenum, and thus extending to the bladder. The causative agent may be the B. coli, streptococci, typhoid, cholera, pneumonia and possibly the influenza bacilli. Having gained access, further developments depend upon various circumstances; for instance the kind and virulence of the bacteria, the general health and resistance of the individual, and whether the gall bladder is already the seat of any pathological condition such as one due to previous attacks of infection or gall stones. Depending upon these circumstances there may be developed any one of the following forms of cholecystitis:

1.—Catarrhal.
2.—Fibrinous.
3.—Suppurative.

CATARRHAL CHOLECYSTITIS.

In this form one finds the changes in the mucous membrane which occur in catarrhal processes elsewhere. As a result of the thickening of the lining, involving as it does the bile ducts also, the drainage is impaired. Because of this, a part of the mucus secreted, is retained, together with what bile there may be present. The watery elements are absorbed, and a thick glutinous mass remains. Particles of the mucus may become inspissated. Occasionally such a piece may engage in the duct, and the effort made to expel it causes symptoms closely simulating those present during the expulsion of a gall stone. To these hard masses of mucus, biliary pigment, cholesterin crystals and other pieces of mucus may adhere, and the product thus formed is what constitutes a gall stone. Catarrhal cholecystitis thus becomes a necessary precursor of cholelithiasis.

The symptoms of this condition are not very definite, unless the gall stones have formed. Otherwise they are usually evidenced only by symptoms arising from the associated cholangitis.

FIBRINOUS CHOLECYSTITIS.

In this condition there is a development of new tissue elements, beginning as small round cells in any or all of the coats of the viscus. These cells pass through the usual changes that take place in fibrinous inflammation, and in this manner a hyperplasia of some part of the organ is produced. If it is the mucous coat, it becomes over-developed, and in case the bladder is not distended by some secretion or by gall stones,—or even to some extent if it is so distended, the muscular coat is apt also to become hypertrophied. It afterwards contracts, and thus reduces the size of the gall bladder, sometimes to such an extent that its cavity is obliterated. The condition is then spoken of as obliterative inflammation of the gall bladder. If the fibrinous process involves to any extent the serous coat, there are adhesions to surrounding organs and other peritoneal coverings. These adhesions are of the same import as those mentioned when considering peritonitis arising from cholangitis and are apt to produce the same obscure digestive symptoms.

SUPPURATIVE CHOLECYSTITIS.

There are two forms of suppurative cholecystitis.

1.—Simple.

2.—Phlegmonous.

When there is a more or less free secretion of pus from the mucous lining, associated with obstruction of the cystic duct by swelling or gall stone, there is an accumulation in the gall bladder alone, and it is called a simple empyema of the gall bladder. If the obstruction is in the common duct, there is an associated suppurative cholangitis. This seriously complicates the condition, as in this case the pus may be blocked back into the small bile ducts ramifying in the parenchyma of the liver, with the dangers described when speaking of this condition resultant from cholangitis alone.

Symptomatology:—These diseases are usually though not always preceded by hepatic colic. (40 out of 51 cases). At first when pus begins to form there may be no marked constitutional symptoms. Whether fever arises or not depends upon whether the cystic duct is involved. If the process is confined to the gall bladder, not even extending down deeply into its neck, there is not apt to be fever, for the reason that in the walls of the bladder itself there are no lymphatics present to absorb the products of pus formation. If however, the disease extends into the neck and into the duct then fever is a marked symptom, for in these places lymphatics are prominent. The fever, if present, is apt to be very irregular in its manifestations, chills, temperature and sweating coming on at varying intervals. There is generally some pain, although this is sometimes not very marked, at other times it is extremely severe. There is malaise, loss of appetite and flesh, local tenderness, and there may be a tumor which can be felt upon palpation if the abdominal walls are not too thick. Icterus is sometimes present, but only when there is some occlusion of the common duct, either from swelling of its lining, or from the presence of a gall stone. At other times no icterus is noticeable.

Diagnosis:—If gall stone colic or some of the bacterial diseases mentioned in the etiology of cholecystitis have preceded a condition where there is malaise, possibly slight jaundice, irregular fever, some tenderness over gall bladder, which can be palpated, one should think of this condition. Cases with marked pain may have to be differentiated from appendicitis, intestinal obstruction, and localized peritonitis, or from perforation of a gastric or duodenal ulcer. Some cases without very much pain but with fever, may have to be distinguished from malaria, typhoid or tuberculosis. Undoubtedly many cases which in the past have been diagnosed as some such indefinite trouble as bilious fever, gastric fever, etc., were in reality suppurative cholecystitis or cholangitis.

Phlegmonous suppurative cholecystitis is a very rare condition, only a few cases having been reported. It is usually associated with gall stones, though it may arise independently, as from some of the infectious fevers. It consists of a circumscribed abscess of the walls of the gall bladder.

The symptoms are those of acute peritonitis of this region, and are very similar to those of abscess arising from appendicitis, except, as a rule, they are located somewhat higher in the abdomen. However, mistakes in differentiating between the two affections have been made, especially where the gall bladder is displaced downward, or the appendix and cæcum have never descended to their usual location. Occasionally the condition will tend to gangrene, and the symptoms will be so mild that the seriousness of the affection will go unappreciated.

TREATMENT OF INFLAMMATORY AFFECTIONS OF THE BILE TRACT.

This resolves itself into prophylactic and curative. Inasmuch as the catarrhal form is in the large majority of cases secondary to gastroenteritis, care should be taken not to indulge in injudicious eating that will be apt to bring on an attack of that trouble. Eating too much food, too rich food, indigestible food, or food which is too hot, too cold, or too highly spiced, or using drinks that contain a high percentage of alcohol, are liable to act as causative agents. A sedentary occupation does not favor as free drainage from the gall bladder and ducts as does a more active life, thus permitting an infection to more easily travel up from the duodenum.

When an inflammation has made its appearance, extra care should be taken as regards the diet. In the acute form it is better to put the patient to bed and withdraw all food until symptoms begin to abate. Then begin with thin soups and increase the diet very gradually, practically the same as in acute gastritis. Give no solid food until the urine has cleared of bile and the stools are again stained by it. If there is constipation, it should be relieved by mild laxatives or enemata. The idea of giving a so-called cholagogue in cases where there is icterus, expecting it to so thin the bile, or to so change it that it will more easily pass the natural channels, is fallacious. It has been proved by numerous experiments that such agents do not affect the bile to any appreciable extent. Taking water in large amounts will probably have some effect in diluting the bile, the same as it does the other secretions of the body, and thus it may be useful.

In chronic catarrhal affections, a more nutritious diet should be given. It should be chosen according to the digestive capabilities of the individual patient. It is customary to give as little fat as practicable, especially when the flow of bile is at all obstructed. If the inflammation is of the fibrinous nature, the same attention should be given to the diet, and carefully selected remedies according to the indications mentioned below should be given. If such methods do not give satisfactory relief, resort to surgery may be necessary in order to liberate adhesions or relieve obstructions. If pus has formed, some method of drainage must be employed, usually a cholecystostomy. Patients may survive if such operation is not performed, but if they do, convalescence is always prolonged to an indefinite extent, and generally leaves a chronic state of partial invalidism.

Chelidonium 3x:—Congested feeling in hepatic region, with pain under right shoulder blade. Yellow tongue, with bitter taste and desire for acids. Feeling of lassitude and indolence. Pasty stools and yellow urine. Metabolic processes seem to be imperfectly performed, there being a tendency to what has been commonly called biliousness. Frequently some icterus. Headache and melancholia.

Chionanthus 2x:—Especially where inflammatory trouble has come down from the liver. Jaundice is nearly always present when this remedy is indicated. Pain may be slight or severe and is of a colicky nature; generally tenderness. Clay colored stools, saffron colored urine which stains the clothing. Often indigestion. Troubles apt to be caused by alcoholic liquors.

Hydrastis 2x:—Secondary to gastric and duodenal catarrh. Faint, gone feeling in the epigastrium. Eyes and conjunctivae are icteric. Tongue is coated yellow. There is constipation, frequently associated with hæmorrhoids; light colored stools, dark urine. This remedy is very frequently a useful one.

Podophyllum 3x:—This in material doses has been considered a cholagogue. If true, this must be due to an irritant action on the liver and bile ducts. As said before, this cholagogue action is largely imaginary, yet podophyllum in minute doses undoubtedly has a beneficial action on irritated bile ducts. It may be used where there is a so-called biliousness, often accompanied with giddiness, bitter taste and risings of food, which sometimes tastes sour, sometimes bitter. The stools are changeable in appearance and color and are apt to be preceded by some colic. Symptoms worse from 2 to 5 a. m.

Myrica 2x:—Yellow, jaundiced appearance, with itching of the skin. Dull pain in biliary region. Debility and drowsiness. Stools are soft, mushy and light yellow or clay colored. Much gas in the intestine.

Mercurius sol. 3x:—Swelling and distention in hepatic region, with considerable stitching pain. Slight icterus. Ineffectual urging to stool, the stools being greenish and often containing mucus. In suppurative forms.

Cinchona 3x:—Much swelling and pain in liver. Very sensitive to touch. Trouble likely to have been preceded by malaria. Useful in suppurative affections with chill, fever and sweat. No appetite, great prostration. Tympanitis.

Nux vomica 3x:—After alcoholic excesses, with gastritis and duodenitis. Constipation, with frequent ineffectual urging to stool. Yellow coating at base of tongue, possibly slight icterus, bitter taste in mouth.

Kali bichromicum 3x:—Duodenal catarrh with complications of the bile tract. Tongue irregularly coated,—the so-called mapped tongue.

Sulphur 6x:—May be useful in chronic troubles, and in those having a tendency to suppurate. Stitches in region of liver, or pressing pain. Selection must often be made more from the well known constitutional symptoms, than from any especially pertaining to this region.

Natrum sulphuricum 6x:—Such tenderness in this region that walking hurts on account of the jarring. Feeling of tension, interfering with deep breathing. Tight lacing is painful. Dirty appearing tongue.

CHAPTER IV.

CHOLELITHIASIS—GALL STONES.

Concretions, within either the gall bladder or the ducts, are of very frequent occurrence. In people dying from all causes, upon whom post mortems have been held, different observers have found gall stones varying in frequency from 2% to 25%. This wide variation is due to various causes such as diet, occupation and characteristic diseases of the districts in which the different observers lived; the age and sex of the subjects examined are also factors. In this country, it has been claimed that 10% of all people over forty years of age, have gall stones. It certainly is a fact that they are often found at autopsy when there had been no previous evidence of their existence. Although in such cases if attention is given to the history, there probably have existed symptoms of dyspepsia or indigestion.

Cholesterin is the chief and necessary ingredient found in their composition. Other substances are bile pigment, mucus, lime salts and degenerated epithelium. Their color and consistence vary according to the proportion of these ingredients. For instance if they are light colored and soft enough to be easily crushed between the fingers, they consist largely of cholesterin. If they are darker,—either yellowish, brownish, or reddish, they contain larger amounts of bile pigment. If they are very hard it is due to the large amount of lime salts in their structure. Their size also varies from minute grains resembling sand, up to three ounces and a half,—this being the size of the largest one ever described. They may number but one, or from that up to several hundred. In one case 1,754 were reported to have been found.

Etiology :—Much speculation has been indulged in as regards the causation of these concretions. It would seem that all causes seriously considered in modern times, may be grouped into two general classes:

1.—Biliary stasis.

2.—Bacterial infection.

As regards the first of these essentials, a great number of factors may be considered as having some influence. It is an acknowledged fact that women are more liable to this complaint than are men. That stagnation of bile is more apt to be present with them may be accounted for by the facts that they live a less active life, that their clothing offers more constriction around the region of the gall bladder, and that the pressure of the uterus in pregnancy interferes with the biliary excretion. No age is exempt from gall stones, as they have been found in unborn babes; yet the latter half of life is the period when they are more frequent. This can be apparently accounted for by the fact that there is an inclination to take less physical exercise at this time. When found in children, it is probable in most cases that there is some congenital malformation interfering with the free passage of the bile. Those who work at some occupation where they sit a good deal, especially if leaning over a table, as in studying, sewing, or at a work-bench, are more liable to have them, because the position compresses the waist line and thus reduces the bile current. Individuals who have some other ailment, such as cardiac lesions, gout or rheumatism are frequent sufferers. Other explanations have been offered as to the reason sufferers from these complaints are so often affected, but such explanations seem unnecessary because the decreased exercise taken by such invalids could not help but increase bile stagnation, this alone supplying one of the important causes.

Various forms of diet have been accused of being responsible for gall stones. For instance Mayo Robson thinks that a diet poor in nitrogen,—that is one consisting largely of carbohydrates, does not cause as large a formation of glychocholate and taurocholate of soda and that these products act as solvents of cholesterin. Therefore if they are decreased in amount there is apt to be a greater precipitation of cholesterin crystals. As evidences of the correctness of this theory, the idea is put forward that the reason that gouty patients are subject to gall stones, is because it is customary for them to be kept largely on a non-nitrogenous diet. The claim is also made that diabetics never have gall stones because they take such a largely nitrogenous diet. The theory is ingenious, and possibly has something in it, but positive information on the subject is hard to obtain. It has also been said that excessive amounts of fat assist in producing gall stones; but possibly this is because it is likely to have some effect in causing gastrointestinal troubles.

The second essential, bacterial infection, is one that has been considered more especially in recent years. Investigation has shown that bile is sterile, except when there is disease of the gall bladder or the ducts; but when abnormal conditions are found in these places, notably in cholelithiasis, bacteria of some form are practically always present, either in the bile or in the substance of the stone itself. Furthermore, the injecting of bacteria of the proper kind into the gall bladders of the lower animals has resulted in the formation of stones, where provision was made at the same time to cause a greater or less degree of biliary stasis. If this provision were not made, the bacteria passed away with the bile, and no stone formed.

Of the various forms of bacteria, the B. coli communis is the one that has been most frequently found. It will be remembered that this is also the one most often found in cholangitis and cholecystitis. In fact the commonly accepted idea now is, that these conditions must necessarily precede cholelithiasis. Therefore excessive eating, or other

things which would cause a gastro-enteritis, would predispose to gall stones, by assisting in causing the primary
conditions.

Next to the B. coli, the typhoid fever bacillus is most often found. For some time it has been recognized that people who have had typhoid, are more apt to have gall stones
than others. The condition may manifest itself soon after
the fever, or not for many years. In some of the latter
cases examination has revealed the typhoid bacilli in the
stone, usually in the form of a "clump" in the center of
the concretion. The theory has been promulgated that in
certain circumstances they undergo the "clumping" process in the bile, and that this serves as a nucleus to which
the other ingredients may adhere.

Whatever bacteria are present, they must be of a certain
virulence. If they are very virulent, gall stones are not
formed, but a suppurative cholecystitis develops instead.
Therefore in experiments upon animals it has been necessary to reduce by culture methods the virulence of the bacteria, to such a degree that the inflammation of the mucous
membrane will advance only to a catarrhal stage, and not
to the suppurative.

When the above two essentials are present, the concretion may start in any one of various ways. For instance,
a "clump" of bacteria may act as the nucleus. At other
times, some particle of foreign matter serves the purpose.
Probably the most frequent manner is as follows:—epithelial cells which have desquamated as a result of the catarrhal process undergo a form of degeneration resulting
in minute droplets of fat, or myelin. Several of these
droplets coalesce, and to them adhere the other substances
going to the formation of a gall stone. The concretion

thus gradually grows by the force of adhesion, the mucus always present in catarrh assisting in causing this.

Pathology:—The changes occurring in the gall bladder and bile ducts as complications of gall stones, are chiefly of an inflammatory nature, and are therefore described under cholecystitis and cholangitis. There is first a catarrh of the mucous lining. In fact, this precedes the gall stones and acts as a causative agent. However, this condition is sometimes aggravated by the pressure of the stones, combined with an infection by the bacteria that are adhering to their surfaces. As a result of the increased inflammation thus caused, a severer degree of pathology may ensue which will involve the muscular coats, and end in a hyperplasia of tissue elements. As such new tissue becomes older it contracts and in this way causes a material shrinking of the viscus. Associated with this may be a plastic inflammation of the serous coat, causing adhesions to surrounding viscera and tissues. Pressure of a stone on a contracting wall of the gall bladder, occasionally causes an ulcer to form, which in some cases may penetrate all the coats. If adhesions to other organs have formed, the ulcerative process penetrates them, thus allowing the stone to gain access to their cavities. When this occurs it is most frequently into the duodenum, but it may be into the stomach, liver or peritoneal cavity. Instances have been reported where stones have traveled by such process to distant parts, such as the lungs, bronchi, iliac region and genito-urinary organs. Occasionally by traumatism, accompanied by severe infection, a suppurative or phlegmonous inflammation arises, either in the walls of the gall bladder or in other parts to which a stone has burrowed its way. It is also undoubtedly a fact that the irritation produced by a gall stone often results in the development of a carcinoma.

Symptomatology :— People having gall stones may be divided into three classes:

1.—Those who have no symptoms whatever, and in whom gall stones are not suspected.

2.—Those in whom various reflex symptoms are present as a result of the irritation of the lining of the gall bladder by the stones, but still who have no characteristic symptoms. These reflex symptoms may be indefinite in nature. Possibly they consist of a dragging sensation in the hypochondriac, epigastric or præcordial regions; or the pain may be sharp and lancinating, extending in various directions, as under the scapula, to the shoulder, to the groin, or it may be localized around the region of the liver, gall bladder, stomach or heart. Sometimes the pains resemble those of angina pectoris, or there may be neuralgia of various parts, headache or such cutaneous sensations as burning or itching. Indigestion, functional in nature so far as the stomach is concerned, is one of the most frequent reflex symptoms. Undoubtedly many symptoms, as of hyperchlorhydria, are dependent upon the irritation caused by gall stones to the nerves and circulation of the digestive area. Lastly, such mental aberrations as melancholia and mental irritability are sometimes associated with gall stones.

3.—However, the chief interest attaches to the limited few, in whom the severe symptoms of so-called hepatic colic are manifested. These attacks are in most cases caused by a stone which has been lodging in the gall bladder, and in some way engages in the ducts to the intestine and tries to pass through them. A typical attack of gall stone colic generally presents the following symptoms:

1.—Pain. Severe pain commences possibly unheralded, at other times preceded by some ill-defined distress about the epigastric region. It is mostly felt directly over the gall bladder, but also involves the entire hepatic region, front and back, and often radiates in other directions. It is colicky in nature, continuous, and very severe, causing the sufferer to cry, moan and writhe in agony. Women who have borne children say that the pain of gall stone colic is much worse than that of parturition. These pains seem to be due to the spastic contraction of the gall bladder and ducts. The entire hepatic area is very sensitive to pressure, and sometimes the dullness is increased in extent. The colic ceases either when the stone passes through into the duodenum, drops back into the gall bladder, or when the duct becomes dilated, and so does not continue in its spastic contraction.

2.—Vomiting. This generally appears a little after the pain. At first it consists of the stomach contents, but later, provided the ductus communis choledochus is not obstructed it may contain bile. The effort at vomiting sometimes seems to help force the stone either into the intestine, or back into the bladder. When this occurs the pain is apt to stop suddenly during an attack of vomiting.

3.—Jaundice. This may appear several hours after an attack of hepatic colic has started, provided the stone has lodged for any length of time in the common duct. Or it may not show until after the attack has ceased. The degree of jaundice developed depends upon the period of time the common duct was obstructed. It may be such a slight tinge that it can only be detected by the closest scrutiny, and shows only in the conjunctivæ, or so pronounced that the entire surface of the body becomes saffron colored. Its duration may be only transient, or persist for months. In the latter case, it indicates that obstruction of the common duct still continues. Jaundice when caused by gall stones is always accompanied by the presence of bile pigment in the urine, which may cause it to become very yellow or almost black in color. At the same time, the bile being prevented from gaining access to the intestine, the fæces lose their natural appearance, and become grayish or clay colored. It must not be thought however that jaundice appears in all cases of gall stone colic, or even in a majority of them. Probably in at least half the cases there can be found no traces of such condition.

4.—Fever. If the attack is long continued, fever often develops, sometimes only to a slight extent, at other times becoming quite high. There is a question as to whether it is due to absorption of bile or to traumatism of the nerve centres. It usually subsides quickly upon the cessation of the pain.

Besides the above important or characteristic symptoms, others of a more general nature are usually present to a greater or less extent. These may be a loss of appetite, frequently increased thirst, a feeling of weakness, irregularity of the heart's action and possibly symptoms of collapse.

The complications and sequelæ which may develop as a result of gall stones may be arranged in two groups:

1.—Those arising when the stone or stones remain in the gall bladder or ducts.

2.—Those arising during the process of escape from these usual confines, or after they have escaped.

If a stone becomes lodged in the cystic duct and oc. cludes it, the bile remaining in the gall bladder is usually absorbed, and the walls contract on the remaining stones if there be any. This may cause a most severe inflammation, resulting in adhesions to surrounding organs, or in the development of an empyema.

If the stone passes to the common duct, and remains there, it causes absorption of bile. If obstruction is complete, a condition of cholæmia develops, in which boils are apt to form on any part of the body, and there is a great tendency toward hæmorrhage upon the slightest injury. This tendency to hæmorrhage seriously interferes with any operative plans which might be considered for relief of the condition. Hydrops of the gall bladder may be present, or if bacteria of the proper kind and virulence are in ts cavity, suppurative cholecystitis will ensue. Owing to the traumatism of the stone on the walls of the ducts, an ulcer may form, which will later contract and leave a stricture, seriously interfering with the passage of bile, and especially of another stone should one attempt to pass at a later date. On the other hand, the ulcer may penetrate the walls, allowing the escape of the stone or of infected bile into the peritoneal cavity, providing protective adhesions have not formed. By means of such adhesions and ulceration through the walls of the duodenum, a large stone may gain access there, and becoming lodged somewhere in the intestine, cause a form of ileus.

Diagnosis:—The symptoms of atypical cases of gall stone colic may simulate almost any abdominal affection. The condition has been confounded with appendicitis, renal colic, pancreatitis, pancreatic calculus, gastric and duodenal ulcer, pyloric cancer, angina pectoris, lead colic, locomotor ataxia, gastralgia, acute indigestion, hysteria, pneumonia, pleurisy and certain forms of intradominal herniæ. This is too long a list to attempt a differential diagnosis, but the symptoms of these conditions should be considered in any doubtful case.

The diagnosis of gall stone colic must ordinarily be made where there is a paroxysmal attack of severe pain, starting in the region of the gall bladder, radiating over the abdomen and to the back and right scapula, accompanied by vomiting. If during such an attack jaundice develops, or if the urine upon examination contains an abnormal amount of bile pigment, or the stools become clay colored, the diagnosis is almost positive, although one should not ordinarily wait for these symptoms before making a decision. Extreme tenderness on a line from the ninth costal cartilage to the umbilicus is almost as diagnostic of gall stones, as tenderness at McBurney's point is indicative of appendicitis.

Treatment:—Inasmuch as catarrhal cholecystitis is probably a necessary precursor of cholelithiasis, the treatment of the former trouble constitutes prophylactic treatment. In fact, so far as remedial measures of a medical nature are concerned, such treatment is all that is of any apparent value. Any attempt to give remedies with the purpose of dissolving stones that have formed in the gall bladder is manifestly absurd and need not be considered.

During an attack of hepatic colic, palliative measures are very necessary. The application of moist heat is often of some value. Emptying the stomach thoroughly by means of the stomach tube may be beneficial, although the vomiting that is generally present will do this in most cases. Many times the administration of some opiate is necessary. Morphia sulphate hypodermically will answer the purpose most satisfactorily. ¼ grain at least is necessary, and sometimes more than that amount. Ordinarily it is best to administer that quantity and wait from fifteen minutes to half hour. If relief is not apparent by that time a dose of from $\frac{1}{8}$ to $\frac{1}{4}$ grain may be added. In cases that have taken the drug repeatedly for this condition, and so have to some extent become accustomed to it, one can with safety give a larger initial dose. It is important to be careful however and not give a larger amount than necessary, because if the stone suddenly passes from the duct an alarming and even dangerous condition may arise from such over dosage. Many times it does well to add atropia sulphate to the morphia, not only for the reasons that it is usually added, but also because of its well known action in producing a relaxation of circular muscle fibres. In this case, if it so acts upon the fibres of the bile ducts, they will to some extent dilate, and the concretion can the more easily pass through to the intestine. After a few hours, if the effects of the morphia begin to pass away, and the pain continues, the dose should be repeated. Chloroform or ether may be used to relieve the excruciating pain, although they are not often necessary.

The question often arises as to whether it is the part of wisdom to resort to surgery in cases of cholelithiasis. In recent years this has been done much more frequently than formerly. As in all other conditions conservatism seems the better way. If frequent attacks of the pain are producing too great suffering, or if the presence of gall stones is giving rise to such reflex trouble, digestive or otherwise, that the health is impaired, it is undoubtedly wise to operate. If they have become lodged in one of the ducts, or if some such complication as suppurative cholangitis or chcolecystitis has arisen, operation should be performed. The best method of operation depends considerably upon circumstances and conditions. In the majority of cases cholecystostomy will give satisfactory results. At other times cholecystectomy will be needed.

CHAPTER V.

TUMORS OF THE GALL BLADDER AND BILE DUCTS.

Considering enlargements of the gall bladder and ducts in the broadest sense, they may be divided into three classes:

1.—Distentions.

2.—Hypertrophies.

3.—Neoplasms.

If the common duct becomes obstructed by a calculus, a stricture or pressure from external causes, the gall bladder and also the ducts above the obstruction may be temporarily distended with bile. However this is not apt to last very long, for, although the hepatic cells continue to secrete the bile it is easily absorbed by the lymphatics, and thus enters the blood. At the same time the mucous lining of the gall bladder and ducts, seemingly irritated by the stagnating contents and the bacteria present, quite frequently begins to send forth an excretion which replaces the bile. This causes a different kind of distention. The excretion may be mucus, in which case the condition is called hydrops of the gall bladder; or pus may form, and then it is called empyema of the gall bladder or suppurative cholecystis. The extent to which a gall bladder may be distended varies widely. Cases of hydrops have been reported where the entire abdomen became invaded, and in which the condition has been mistaken for ovarian cyst. Besides being distended with bile, mucus and pus, a gall bladder may contain so many calculi that it becomes considerably enlarged. Another form of distention, very rare in this country but comparatively frequent in some places, is an hydatid cyst, due to the presence of a certain form of parasite.

By hypertrophy is meant the thickening which takes place as a result of the inflammatory process. Such a condition, though hardly what is commonly considered as a tumor, yet forms a hard resistant mass which upon palpation quite closely resembles a new growth.

Of the true neoplasms carcinoma is by far the most common one present. It may be primary, in which case it is nearly always caused by the irritation of gall stones, or it may be secondary. If the latter it may owe its existence in the gall bladder to metastases from other parts, or to extension by contiguity from surrounding organs. The organs from which it is most apt to extend are the stomach, liver, colon and pancreas.

Symptoms:—Beginning with sensations of discomfort and fullness in the region of the gall bladder, there soon arises more decided pain. The pain extends through the epigastrium, hypogastrium and frequently to the right side and infrascapular region. In favorable subjects a swelling can soon be palpated. It is hard to the touch, not very sensitive, and descends with inspiration. Later it may become nodular and adherent. It usually in the course of time involves the liver, stomach, duodenum, pancreas and colon. Glandular enlargements and peritoneal complications often develop, sometimes giving rise to ascites. In about half the cases the hepatic or common ducts become involved, and then there is more or less icterus. If complicated with cholelithiasis there are apt to be paroxysmal attacks, resembling malaria. That is, there will be chills, fever and perspiration, quite often coming on at regular intervals. After such attacks, there will be an increase of the jaundice. At the time of a paroxysm there is generally an aggravation of the pain.

Other neoplasms of the gall bladder are so rare that no attempt will be made to describe such growths. Sarcomata have been reported; also papillomata and adenomata.

Diagnosis:—Tumors of this region are notably difficult to diagnose. Tumors of the gall bladder, pylorus, pancreas, intestine, liver, suprarenal capsule or right kidney all possess features of similarity. However, if there is a history of gall stone colic, perhaps some jaundice and a palpable tumor on a line between the costal cartilage on the right side and the umbilicus, it is fair to presume that there is a tumor of the gall bladder, probably a cancer. Sometimes a sulcus may be detected between it and the liver. The growth is then generally nodular, hard and of the general shape of the gall bladder. In case a positive diagnosis can not be made, a small exploratory incision may be done with comparative safety.

Treatment:—The medical treatment is simply palliative. It consists in keeping up the patient's nutrition as well as possible by means of diet selected to meet digestive indications, and relief of pain. Remedies selected for such purpose may be sufficient in the earlier stages, but morphia will ultimately have to be employed in most cases.

If the diagnosis is made early, while the process is still confined to the gall bladder, surgery may be employed and an attempt made to eradicate the trouble. Usually however, when it has advanced far enough to be diagnosed, it has extended beyond the gall bladder, and complete removal can not be effected.

Part V.—Diseases of the Liver.

CHAPTER I.

PERI-HEPATITIS.

Definition:—By peri-hepatitis is meant, not an inflammation of the peritoneal covering of the liver, but of the fibrous coat, or so-called Glisson's capsule.

Etiology:—The causes which give rise to this trouble are mechanical such as pressure by corsets and tight clothing, or injuries that may be received from blows, severe jars or falling. The condition may also arise by extension, from peritoneal inflammation originating in the gall bladder, or from a gastric ulcer, and it may be from an extension of a pleuritis which has passed through the diaphragm. Diseases starting within the liver, such as cirrhosis, abscess, syphilis, echinococcus and cancer may produce inflammatory changes in Glisson's capsule if they affect the connective tissue of the liver. The trabeculæ of this connective tissue extending to the surface of the organ, constitutes the capsule.

Pathology:—There is a thickening of the fibrous coat, which may be slight in extent, or may increase to 10 millimeters. When it progresses to this latter thickness, contraction occurs and a compression of the liver substance ensues. This may advance to such a degree as to simulate cirrhosis, even giving rise to ascites and other symptoms of that disease, and if the inflammation extends to the trabeculæ in the substance of the liver, real cirrhosis may be produced.

247

Symptoms:—These may be absent, for a time at least. In time the peritoneal covering of .Glisson's capsule becomes affected to an extent sufficient to cause adhesions to surrounding organs. If the capsule thickens enough to cause contraction of the liver, there are symptoms very similar to those present in cirrhosis. In the acute form there may be some pain and tenderness in the hepatic region. If this be present, it is made worse by pressure, as when lying on the affected side, or by deep breathing The pain is sharp and lancinating as in peritonitis. Palpation and percussion are difficult because of the tenderness. As in many cases the condition is an extension from some other trouble, the symptoms due to the peri-hepatitis are apt to be overshadowed by those of the primary disease.

Diagnosis:—The pain and tenderness seems of a more lancinating character than when due to disease of the substance of the liver, and when the liver itself is diseased there is not apt to be as much distress caused by pressure. The pain is also more diffuse and radiates to the scapular region. It is less violent than when due to gall stone colic, and is longer in duration.

Treatment:—Rest in the most comfortable position should be insisted upon. In the early stage of the acute form, an ice bag may be applied over the hepatic region, to be followed later by hot applications or the Priessnitz.

Arnica 3x:—If the trouble was caused by an injury or a jar. There is a sore bruised feeling, often associated with some nausea.

Aconite 3x:—In an acute attack commencing with chill, fever and great arterial excitement.

Bryonia 3x:—The most frequent symptoms present are a lancinating pain, with some fever; pain aggravated by movement or pressure.

If pain becomes extremely severe, morphia may be needed. When it is given, best results will be obtained by hypodermic injections.

CHAPTER II.

HYPERÆMIA OF THE LIVER.

The liver, being a very vascular organ, with vessel walls that are thin and distensible, is subject to wide variations in the amount of blood contained in it at different times. Even in a healthy liver, during the period of functional activity,—that is during the period of digestion,—the supply of blood is increased sufficiently to materially enlarge the organ. Besides the great number and distensibility of the vessels and the compressibility of the parenchyma, the blood in the hepatic veins, flowing as it does directly into the inferior vena cava, may be delayed at this point, as the current in this vessel is greatly influenced by changes in intra-thoracic pressure and by the action and integrity of the heart. For this reason not only disease of the liver, but exercise, position, tightness of clothing and heart disease may, through their effect on the circulation, have a bearing upon the amount of blood contained in the organ under consideration. The left lobe is subject to greater changes than the right, because the latter is to an extent compressed by the ribs so that enlargement is made more difficult.

When caused by diseased conditions, hyperæmia of the liver may be of two kinds:

1.—Active.
2.—Passive.

Active hyperæmia is most often produced by causes pertaining to the digestive system. Eating even a normal amount of food causes some increase in the amount of blood contained in the viscus. If an excessive amount be taken, the increase becomes so great as to be pathologic; therefore gourmands are especially liable to hyperæmia. Certain articles of food and drink have more effect than others, alcohol being especially active, as well as coffee, spices and other stimulating substances. Contusions, the exanthemata, and certain infectious fevers, especially typhoid and malaria, also have some effect in causing the condition. Menstruation may produce it, especially if there be some sudden disturbance of the function, as by cold. Neoplasms, parasites and other diseases of the liver itself may result in acute congestion, although such conditions are more apt to have an influence in causing the passive variety.

Pathology:—So long as the condition is limited to active hyperæmia alone, the increased amount of blood, with enlarged vessels and compression, constitute the only changes present, but if the attacks are frequently repeated or continuously present, the changes will begin to appear, which will later be considered under the subject of cirrhosis.

Symptomatology:—Inasmuch as active hyperæmia is so frequently associated with other conditions, such as various digestive troubles, fevers and auto-intoxication, it is not always easy to distinguish the symptoms due to this trouble alone. There is generally a sensation of pressure and fullness in the hepatic region, which may even become a severe pain, especially during the period of digestive activity. There is flatulence and pyrosis, with a feeling of vertigo and mental depression. If the hyperæmia is severe, there may be enough swelling to cause compression of the bile ducts, with slight jaundice. In such a severe type there will probably be some fever. Palpation and percussion will give evidence of enlargement, which is especially marked in the left lobe, and its presence may be easily detected because it is easy of access.

Diagnosis:—It is often difficult to diagnosticate this affection from other hypertrophic condition of the liver, until time has been taken to watch the effect of treatment. If the above symptoms are present, but improve promptly upon instituting proper regimen and treatment, it is fair to presume that no further pathological conditions have occurred in the hepatic parenchyma; but if the condition has lasted any length of time, without material change in the symptoms or the findings upon physical examination, it is probable that some other trouble is present.

Treatment:—This depends to some extent upon the underlying cause. For instance, if the hyperæmia is due to some infectious disease, the treatment for that disease is of chief importance; if due to miasmatic affections, relief may depend upon removal from the tropical country where contracted. Traumatic hyperæmia demands rest and suitable local applications. In by far the greater number of cases, dietetic errors are responsible, and a correction of such habits is necessary. Even in cases not dependent upon incorrect eating, the diet should be regulated so as to reduce as far as possible the physiological hyperæmia which follows the taking of food. Especial care should be exercised to eliminate articles which stimulate action of the liver. Such articles are alcohol and condiments like pepper, mustard and spices. It is also better to reduce considerably the amount of fat, sugar and salt.

Fresh vegetables and fruits should be allowed freely, unless for special reasons they disagree, for the purpose of helping to overcome the constipation which is generally a factor. For the same reason water should be freely taken. Laxatives may be demanded in some cases, partly to reduce intra-abdominal tension by removing the intestinal contents, thus allowing the blood to circulate more freely; also to prevent putrefactive processes in the intestine giving rise to toxins, which being carried to the liver by the portal vein, act as irritants upon the organ. Either saline or vegetable evacuants may be employed, but care should be exercised that they may not be used strong enough or too often, so as to act as irritants upon the liver. Enemata may be employed in place of laxatives, or possibly by care in diet and general hygiene it will be possible to get along without resorting to either of these means.

Nux vomica 3x:—When caused by overeating, and especially by excessive use of alcohol, strong condiments and coffee. Liver is sore and indurated, there is some tenderness in hepatic region. Constipation, fullness in the head, possibly slight icterus.

China 1x:—After an attack of malaria. There is apt to be considerable jaundice, loss of appetite, weakness. Liver enlarged and sensitive. For a time it may be better to resort to quinine in material doses.

Chelidonium 2x:—Another remedy which is often useful after malaria. There is a feeling of fullness in right side, and especially of pain under the right shoulder blade.

Podophyllum 3x:—Attended with evidences of gastro-duodenal and bile tract trouble. Icteric appearance of eyes, coated tongue, changeable stool, tenderness and enlargement of the liver.

Lycopodium 6x:—Much flatulence, constipation, prostrated condition; apt to have been history of having taken strong medicines, especially cathartics.

Mercurius sol. 3x:—Large flabby tongue, bad taste, congested feeling, patient worse at night.

Arnica 3x:—Following such injuries as falls, contusions or strains.

Bryonia 3x:—Cases may be severe enough to cause some fever, with much thirst, dry coated tongue, constipation, tenderness especially upon moving and stitching pains in the side.

CHAPTER III.

PASSIVE HYPERÆMIA OF THE LIVER.

Etiology:—The most frequent cause of passive congestion of the liver is cardiac insufficiency. This may be due to diseases of the orifices of the heart, to myocarditis or to fatty degeneration. Chronic bronchitis, pleural adhesions, emphysema or contraction of lung tissue, by offering obstruction to the blood propelled by the right side of the heart, may cause sufficient delay of blood in the inferior vena cava to offer obstruction to the hepatic veins. There may be deformities of the spinal column, tumors or pleural exudates, which, by pressure upon this vessel produce the same result. Finally, causes acting from within the liver, such as cicatricial contraction where there have been abscesses, or thrombotic narrowing of veins, may interfere with a free passage of blood from the organ. Such causes, however, and also tight lacing, are more apt to cause localized areas of hyperæmia.

Pathology:—Dilatation occurs, first of the hepatic veins, then of the venous radicles and finally of the central venules of the lobules. Dilatations of these veins cause compression of hepatic tissue, which later leads to atrophy. Sometimes the cells in the center of the lobules become filled with brown pigment, and those near the periphery become fatty. As the trabeculæ of the liver become more atrophied, the walls of the vessels approach each other until they come in contact. When this stage is reached, new connective tissue infiltration may take place between the lobules, and new bile channels may form. This proliferation or formation of new tissue is followed by contraction. After death, in a case of this kind, the veins and capillaries may empty themselves of blood, and thus the size of the liver be reduced, so that a liver which before death could be detected as being enlarged, may at post mortem be but little if at all larger than normal.

Symptomatology :—As this disease always follows disease of some other organ, especially of the heart or lungs, the symptoms of this other affection are also present. The congestion of the liver always develops slowly. As a result, symptoms are apt to be absent for some time, and even when enlargement is quite noticeable upon physical examination, subjective symptoms may not be present. Upon their appearance they differ considerably, but there is generally a feeling of fulness in the epigastrium or on the right side. This sensation is worse after eating when the above mentioned physiological congestion is present. Various dyspeptic symptoms are apt to exist. Icterus of a very mild nature may be discovered, if careful examination be made for it. Ascites may be present to some extent, its intensity depending not so much upon the severity of the congestion as upon the individuality of the patient. Some livers seem to act as a sponge and by holding large amounts of blood which the heart cannot handle, relieve it somewhat. In other cases the liver does not act as such a safety valve, and as' soon as it becomes slightly distended with blood, it squeezes out the watery elements into the peritoneal cavity in the form of ascites.

By palpation and percussion the liver may be detected beyond its usual limits. The surface feels hard and smooth, the margin rounded, extending perhaps to the umbilicus or even lower. If the hyperæmia is due to tricuspid insufficiency, systolic pulsations of the liver may be felt, if the entire hand is laid flatly over its surface. This is due to regurgitation of blood into the inferior vena cava and thence into the hepatic veins. In some cases a development of new connective tissue will take place, which in time undergoes retraction. The liver then becomes atrophied.

Diagnosis:—The one identifying feature in differentiating congestion of the liver from other affections in which the organ is enlarged, is that in this condition its size varies, depending upon the state of the circulation at the time of the examination. For instance exercise, or the position occupied by the patient with its resulting effect upon the circulation, materially influences the amount of blood in the organ, and therefore its size. Likewise on different days, or even at different hours of the same day, there may be quite a change in the outline of the liver.

Treatment:—This is primarily a treatment of the circulatory condition which gives rise to the trouble. For the liver complication itself, a diet free from alcohol and such other irritating articles as mentioned under the subject of active hyperæmia should be prescribed. The amount of food usually needs restriction. Be careful not to let the diet reach such a low point that malnutrition will take place, as this will reduce the strength of the heart muscle, and be likely to still further aggravate the trouble. Free evacuation of the bowels should be encouraged to reduce intra-abdominal tension and also to prevent the absorption of irritating toxins which are liable to be carried from the intestine to the liver. If hepatic pain is present, hot applications will give some relief. If there is sufficient ascites to cause trouble, it should be relieved by diet, and medication if possible, if not, then by abdominal paracentesis. This latter operation relieves some of the impediment to the circulation of the blood through the abdominal cavity, and thus lessens the work which the heart has to perform. If remedies are necessary for the treatment of the hepatic condition itself, they will usually be the ones mentioned when considering active hyperæmia of the liver.

CHAPTER IV.

ACUTE HEPATITIS.

Acute hepatitis may be divided into three kinds:

1.—Acute parenchymatous hepatitis.
2.—Acute atrophy of the liver.
3.—Acute interstitial hepatitis.

ACUTE PARENCHYMATOUS HEPATITIS.

Etiology:—This is very often a sequel to some of the infectious diseases, especially malaria, typhoid, erysipelas, septicæmia, puerperal fever, pneumonia and dysentery. In some of these diseases, especially malaria, sepsis and typhoid, the pathological organisms may be found in the liver. It is not thought however that these organisms cause the inflammation by their local presence, but rather that it is caused by chemical poisons generated in other parts of the body and transported to the liver by the blood current. The disease is especially rife in the torrid zones, due no doubt to the prevalence of malaria and dysentery in these places, though some who go to warm climates from the higher latitudes may have the trouble without such a causative disease preceding, especially during the first or second year of their residence. It has been found that if they eat sparingly, particularly of animal foods, and refrain from alcoholic drinks, they are much less apt to be attacked. Besides the poisons produced by infectious organisms, certain others such as chloroform, phosphorus and some of the mushroom fungi may cause acute parenchymatous hepatitis. Alcohol is a very potent agent in its causation.

Pathology:—The hepatic cells appear cloudy and contain granulations which at first are albumen, but later change to fat. The cells may be swollen, in this way somewhat enlarging the liver. In severe cases especially those due to sepsis, the trabeculæ enclosing the cells become degenerated so that the cells are loosened. They then become indistinct, necrosis occurs, and the nuclei and protoplasm do not stain as readily as normally. When due to phosphorus poisoning, a marked fatty degeneration takes place. In the form usually found in the tropics, the liver is enlarged and contains much blood. Grayish foci, more or less softened permeate its substance. Later these foci become yellow, and finally undergo atrophic changes. These changes are probably due to intestinal ptomaines which are carried to the liver and act as irritants.

Symptomatology:—There is usually vomiting, diarrhœa, and pain in the region of the liver. There may be but mild fever, or in some cases there are chills and high fever. Often there is mild icterus, a feeling of pressure under the margin of the ribs, pain in the right shoulder and impeded respiration. The liver may be but slightly enlarged, or it may reach several inches below the costal margin. As it is usually a sequel to some other affection the symptoms of such primary disease are apt to so over- shadow the hepatitis that in many cases it is overlooked, at least in the early stages.

Prognosis:—The first attack usually terminates favor- ably in from eight to fourteen days. However, it predis- poses to later attacks, which are generally more severe and longer lasting, and which may terminate in abscess or some form of degeneration with fatal outcome.

Treatment:—The methods of treating this trouble, acute interstial hepatitis and abscess of the liver will be con- sidered together.

ACUTE ATROPHY OF THE LIVER.

Although this is nearly always a sequel to acute par- enchymatous hepatitis, yet it possesses characteristics dis- tinguishing it from the simple form of that disease, suf- ficient to merit separate study.

Etiology:—It is quite a rare disease. It is more fre- quent in the warmer climates, and is most often found in young women during pregnancy. It is also occasionally found in children. It has been demonstrated that cer- tain of the chemical poisons such as phosphorus, alcohol, arsenic, lead and antimony may act as causative factors. Ptomaines resulting from intestinal putrefaction may also produce the condition. It has been known to follow some of the infectious diseases, in fact the same ones that cause acute parenchymatous hepatitis.

Pathology:—Whatever its exciting cause, its first man- ifestation is usually a catarrhal cholangitis which travels up into the fine bile ducts of the liver. Reaching the parenchyma of the liver in the form of an inflammation, atrophy of an acute form develops. The size of the liver is much reduced, particularly the left lobe. The weight of the organ may not be more than half the normal. It becomes flattened, folded on itself and located near the spinal column. It is soft in consistence, and the color changes to yellow, which in many instances is intermixed with red. This latter may exist only as small foci, or it may constitute the chief substance, so that the yellow portions appear as foci. The red portions are tougher than the yellow, and when a section is cut, the red protrudes beyond the surface. The lobules are indistinct in outline, and the cells comprising them are less degenerated near the center than at the periphery. Sometimes the degeneration is granular, at other times it is fatty. At first the capillary blood vessels are not affected, but later they become brittle and perish, as do also the bile capillaries. The connective tissue is sometimes increased in amount. The cubical epithelia lining the bile passages are also increased in numbers, sometimes to such an extent that irregularly shaped lobules are formed of them, surrounded by connective tissue. These epithelial cells may undergo certain changes, and to some extent perform the functions of hepatic cells, in this manner improving the condition of the patient. Crystals of tyrosin are found in the urine of individuals suffering from this disease. The process of their formation is unknown. Besides the changes found in the liver itself, there are apt to be diseased conditions of other organs. The epithelium of the kidneys, the muscle fibres of the heart, and sometimes the general muscular system, become icteric and granular, and may undergo fatty degeneration. In the stomach and intestine, the epithelial and glandular cells undergo the same changes, as does also the bronchial epithelium. The spleen increases in size, and the follicular and mesenteric glands enlarge. Ecchymotic spots appear on serous membranes, the skin and the digestive and urinary passages. A marked anæmia is present in all cases.

Symptomatology :—Usually there is a prodromal stage which very closely resembles acute catarrhal cholangitis. It begins with evidence of acute gastro-enteritis, followed in a few days, or weeks, by a mild icterus. During this stage there is apparently a stasis of bile, with the resulting highly colored urine and clay colored stools. The liver is somewhat enlarged because either of biliary stasis or of swelling of the hepatic cells. If caused by phosphorus poisoning, the swelling is more marked than when the disease is produced by other causes. The second stage may be reached in a day or two, or it may take several weeks, but when it does appear, it generally comes on suddenly. There are then pronounced cerebral symptoms, vomiting, hæmorrhages, urinary changes, fever, decreased size of the liver, and pain both in this organ and in the spleen. There may be stupor, delirium, mania or convulsions. The vomited matter is slimy and bloody and often contains bile. There is generally constipation. The hæmorrhages may be from the stomach, intestines, urinary tract or nose, or may present as an ecchymosis. The most characteristic change in the urine is the presence of leucin and tyrosin. There are also apt to be albumen, tube casts, epithelium, bile pigment, sarcolactic acid and albumose. The urea is decreased and the uric acid sometimes increased, especially in favorable cases. The temperature may rise during the prodromal stage; in the beginning of the second stage it is normal, and later becomes sub-normal. Pain is not a very prominent symptom, but there may be a feeling of fulness or even quite severe pain in the hepatic region, and there is usually some headache. The size of the liver rapidly decreases, and may become so small and flaccid that it cannot be palpated. At this time there is much tenderness.

Diagnosis:—When in an icteric subject pronounced cerebral symptoms appear, one should think of acute yellow atrophy, although of course these symptoms may be present in the infectious diseases mentioned as frequently causing this trouble, even where it is not developing. If, however, in addition to the icterus and the cerebral symptoms, there is absence of fever and a marked decrease in the size of the liver, and leucin and tyrosin can be found in the urine, acute yellow atrophy of the liver may be considered as existing.

Prognosis:—In nearly all cases death results. It has been said that 30% of all cases terminate fatally between the fifth and fourteenth day, and 30% of the remainder before the fifth week. A few cases run from several weeks to several months, and exceptionally recovery takes place because of the cubical cells of the bile passages taking on the functions of the liver cells, as mentioned in the pathology.

Treatment:—If in every case of catarrhal cholangitis with icterus the treatment mentioned under that head were carefully carried out, there would be fewer cases of acute yellow atrophy. Especial attention should be given to clearing out the intestinal tract, and thus preventing absorption of toxic products from this source, as it is now believed that such absorption is important in causing the trouble. When the symptoms of the second stage are ushered in, not much benefit can be obtained from any treatment. Rest and light diet should be employed, attention given to the bowels and the case treated symptomatically. Phosphorus seems eminently homœopathic to the trouble when it has not been caused by this agent. In material doses it can certainly cause symptoms similar to the ones present in this disease. It has often been prescribed in the trouble, but seemingly without much benefit.

ACUTE INTERSTITIAL HEPATITIS.

A hyperplasia of connective tissue has been mentioned as occurring in both acute parenchymatous hepatitis and acute yellow atrophy. It is sometimes found without the other processes being present, or possibly the former one is present but to a less noticeable extent than are changes in the interstitial tissues. Such cases are called acute interstitial hepatitis or acute cirrhosis.

The causes are the same as for the parenchymatous form, and the symptoms are also very similar. Possibly there is a little more icterus, and the illness is not quite so acute, often lasting several weeks or even months. When due to syphilis or malaria it is more acute at first, but finally merges into the chronic type.

As the causes and symptoms are so similar to those of the parenchymatous form the treatment should also be practically the same. As these diseases, like abscess of the liver are all of an inflammatory nature, it seems more appropriate to wait until after considering abscess before taking up the question of treatment.

CHAPTER V.

ABSCESS OF THE LIVER.

An abscess located in the liver, as elsewhere, must have as its immediate cause infection by some pus forming bacteria. In this case the most common varieties are streptococci, bacilli coli, and pneumococci. The parasites of malaria, actinomycosis and certain flaggelated organisms have also been found in these cases. Depending upon the manner in which the organisms gain access to the liver, abscesses of this organ may be divided into—

1.—Primary.

2.—Secondary.

By primary are meant those which are caused by traumatism or by a direct extension through ulcerative processes from contiguous organs. The most common examples of this kind are those arising from ulcers of the gall bladder, bile ducts, stomach and duodenum. The upward passage of the infection from the intestine by means of the bile ducts also comes under this head.

Secondary abscesses are more frequent than are the primary. In this form the infection reaches the liver by means of the blood current. It may do this by any one of three different routes:

1.—From the general system through the hepatic artery.

2.—Through the branches of the portal vein.

3.—By means of the hepatic veins.

Infection occurs through the hepatic artery in cases of general pyæmia, purulent endocarditis, purulent bronchitis, suppuration of the lung, and in fact when pus formation is going on in almost any part of the body. It took place more frequently before asepsis and antisepsis were in vogue. It is usually not of very much clinical importance because the primary condition from which it arises is of such a severe type that the liver trouble hardly attracts attention and may not be discovered until autopsy.

Infection through the portal vein derives its greatest importance from the frequency with which the organisms of dysentery are conveyed by this means to the liver, where they give rise to abscesses. This is the most frequent cause of the condition and gives rise to marked and characteristic symptoms. It naturally is seen most frequently in tropical countries, and especially among people who do not exercise care in the selection of their diet. Those who eat too heartily, especially of fatty and nitrogenous foods, and drink too freely of alcoholic beverages are more susceptible than are others, such as those of the Mohammedan religion who are more temperate in their eating and drinking. Besides dysentery, other affections of the intestine permit the transportation of infection to the liver by means of the portal circulation, resulting in abscess. Chief amongst such conditions are suppurative processes about the vermiform appendix and cæcum, and ulcers of the stomach, small intestine or rectum, in fact any part of the abdominal or pelvic viscera drained by branches of the portal vein.

The third method of infection is not thoroughly understood. Apparently when there is suppuration in the lower extremities, pelvis or other parts from which blood passes through the inferior vena cava, sometimes owing to a retrograde blood current, infection gains access to the liver through the hepatic veins. This retrograde movement of the blood is probably always due to some affection of the heart, as, for instance, tricuspid insufficiency.

Pathology:—This varies in the different kinds of abscess. If due to traumatism the parenchyma undergoes disintegration and destruction as a result of the pus formation. Surrounding the abscess, there is a zone of hyperæmia with a resulting pyogenic membrane, which produces an encapsulation. The pus corpuscles make their way between the hepatic cells and in time so affect these cells that they undergo necrosis. If the abscess is near the surface, there is usually an associated peri-hepatitis. If the trouble occurs as a result of infection by means of the hepatic artery or portal vein, multiple abscesses are apt to be present. In size they may be very small or may be as large as two inches in diameter. The pus may be thin, or thick and bloody, or mixed with bile. If the latter, the abscesses appear of a bright yellow color, and surrounding them there may be a green zone, due to the action of bacteria and their products on the liver tissue. In some cases, especially when the infection has occurred from the intestine, and the patient has died very soon, no pus will be found, but instead there will be numerous dark spots. If the infection entered the liver my means of the portal vein, there will be many bacteria and leucocytes in the dilated capillaries of that vein, especially around the vena centralis of the lobules and also between the liver cells. Later the cells undergo disintegration, and within the range of influence of an abscess there will be only fat globules, leucocytes, bacteria and general debris. Tropical abscesses as a rule are single and form more slowly than other varieties. However, they are sometimes extremely abrupt and cause death before pus has time to form.

Symptomatology:—The symptoms may be considered under four heads:

1.—General or constitutional.
2.—Local.
3.—Resulting phenomena displayed in other organs.
4.—Sequelæ.

One of the most important of the constitutional symptoms, is fever. This is practically always present at some stage, and may be of any variety. That is it may be con-

tinued, remittent, intermittent or irregular. Its type and
severity depend upon the location of the abscess and the
kind and virulence of the infection. Usually in the early
inflammatory or pre-suppurative stage it is continued, but
it is sometimes remittent. When pus begins to form, there
is the characteristic irregular fever with chill and high
temperature, followed by sweat and rapid decline to normal or below. In most cases, the fever comes on toward
evening and the perspiration takes place at night. This
intermittent fever resembles to a considerable extent the
fever of sepsis, malaria and tuberculosis, and because of
this fact abscess of the liver may be mistaken for one of
these conditions. Later the fever may subside entirely,
provided the process of suppuration ceases or the abscess
becomes firmly encapsulated. During the fever the pulse
is rapid, and during the interval it often becomes small
and weak. The mind may remain clear, or there may be
a typhoid condition with delirium or coma. Of the symptoms
present in the hepatic region itself, pain is of first importance. At first it may only be a sensation of weight or
compression, generally felt more distinctly in the right
hypochondrium. If the left lobe is affected it may be in
the epigastrium. Later the sensation merges into more
severe pain. Its intensity is greater if the abscess is located near the surface of the liver, and especially if it
involves the capsule. It may then be sharp and lancinating, crushing or boring. It is but seldom throbbing as
in abscess formation elsewhere. It may radiate in different directions, depending considerably upon the location
of the lesion. If the location is deep in the organ where
sensory nerves are absent, there may be but very little
pain. In some cases, no matter where the trouble is located there will be intervals when pain is absent; prob-

ably at these times the suppurative process is remaining quiescent. If the abscess becomes encapsulated as it does sometimes, there will be but slight pain. A very frequent site for pain to be felt is under the shoulder blade, the right one if the abscess is in the right lobe of the liver, the left shoulder if of the left lobe, or in multiple abscesses it may be on both sides. This reflected pain is caused by pressure of the enlarged organ on the phrenic nerve, and as this is derived from the cervical plexus which sends branches to the shoulder and to the upper arm, pain may in some cases be felt in these various locations.

When affected by abscess, the liver becomes considerably enlarged. At first the enlargement is soft, but later it becomes quite hard and firm. The increased size is generally more pronounced in an upward direction, thus pressing against the diaphragm and lung, and also causing an outward bulging of the costal arch on the right side. The intercostal depressions are generally obliterated. If the left lobe is involved there is a marked prominence in the epigastrium, which may entirely cover over the stomach. The lower margin of the organ is generally below its normal location, sometimes a considerable distance.

Symptoms of other parts of the digestive system are generally prominent. As stated in the etiology there are apt to be affections of the stomach and intestine preceding the hepatic abscess. There are many symptoms which are secondary to the abscess, to some extent at least. These are anorexia, bulimia, nausea, vomiting, foul taste and coated tongue. If the liver is much enlarged, taking any amount of food into the stomach will cause an increased feeling of pressure. Abscess involving the covering of the liver will cause a circumscribed peritonitis, and from this, ascites may develop. An effusion may also be present as a result of the cachectic condition which may develop, such effusion sometimes existing as ascites, hydrothorax, anasarca or in various serous sacs. In tropical abscesses, the spleen is not apt to be enlarged, except when malaria has existed. In other forms this organ is often increased in size, and if the suppurative process becomes chronic, amyloid degeneration of the spleen may take place. Myocarditis is sometimes present, with resulting dilatation and weak, irregular action. Abscess of the left lobe may displace the heart upward, and sometimes by direct infection causes a pericarditis. In the blood vessels there may be emboli, resulting in secondary abscesses in the lungs or other organs. Changes in the blood are constant, resulting in anæmia and leucocytosis. The skin is of a cachectic appearance, usually grayish in color. There is not apt to be icterus unless the abscess is complicated with cholangitis. The respiratory organs are usually affected owing to the upward pressure against the diaphragm. There may be dyspnœa and sometimes a dry cough because of pleuritic irritation. Localized pleurisy may be present, sometimes of sufficient intensity to cause empyæma, while from direct invasion of bacteria and the inflammatory process a pneumonia may develop.

As sequelæ of hepatic abscess, amyloid degeneration of the liver itself, or of other organs may mentioned. The most prominent results, however, are caused by the attempt made by the pus to find a place of exit. This may occur in almost any direction, and in pursuing such courses, long sinuous fistulæ may be formed. Adhesions may take place between the liver and the abdominal wall; then the pus may burrow to the surface of the skin and be evacuated. This may be over the liver area, or some distance from it. By the same method the pus may burrow into the lung, and rupturing into a bronchus be expectorated. It may be into the pericardium, where of course it causes death. It may be into the stomach and be vomited, or into the intestine and pass away with the stool, into the peritoneal cavity, into the portal vein or the inferior vena cava or into the right kidney. Cyr, in reporting 563 cases of hepatic abscess, found that 311 found no opening at all. 83 were operated upon, 59 discharged into the lung, 39 into the peritoneal cavity, 31 into the pleural cavity, 13 into the colon, 8 into the stomach or duodenum, 4 into the bile passages, 3 into the inferior vena cava, 2 into the kidney, 2 through the abdominal wall and 1 into the pericardium.

Prognosis:—This depends considerably upon the virulence of the infection, the manner in which it gained access to the liver and the sequelæ which may develop. In tropical countries, abscesses do not seem to be as serious as elsewhere. Abscesses following gall stones and cholangitis quite often terminate favorably after operation or perforation into certain of the cavities, or externally. Those coming on as a result of pyæmia are probably always fatal. Those occurring as a result of traumatism, or of acute infection through the portal vein, often end seriously.

Diagnosis:—In many cases there are other diseased processes present which so fully occupy the attention that hepatic abscess is overlooked. When taking place in pyæmia, septicæmia or acute cholangitis they are usually multiple, and in most cases can only be suspected if there is much pain in the hepatic region. In the case of a person living in a tropical country, or following some disease which is known to act often in a causative manner, a single abscess may generally be diagnosed by the pain, the enlargement in an upward direction, the circumscribed bulging, pain in the shoulder, septic fever, and in some cases by fluctuation. It can generally be differentiated from pleurisy or pneumonia by the bulging of the lower costal margin and the convex area of enlargement upward. If in doubt, one may employ exploratory puncture. A subphrenic abscess may so simulate hepatic abscess that only a close study of the history will enable one to differentiate. Abscess of the left lobe may resemble some stomach trouble, especially cancer. Examination of the stomach contents will generally suffice to distinguish between these troubles. Pulsations of the aorta transmitted through an abscess will sometimes cause one to think of an aortic aneurysm, but the pulsation lacks the expansile quality. The shape and location of the enlarged area are the chief distinctions between abscess of the liver and a gall bladder containing pus. Echinococcus cysts resemble abscess somewhat, but they develop more slowly and without signs of inflammation. Cysts and abscesses of the pancreas can be differentiated by distending the stomach with air. If the pancreas is involved, the stomach will cover it, and if the seat of trouble is in the liver it will be in front of the distended stomach. For the purpose of detecting abscess of the liver and also the kind and virulence of the bacteria causing it, aspiration may be performed. If care be exercised the procedure is comparatively safe, and it renders much assistance in the diagnosis of some cases.

Treatment:—In the treatment of the acute inflammations of the liver, prophylaxis is of great importance. This pertains to diet. Irritating articles or those which may cause gastro-enteritis should be excluded. Drinks containing alcohol are especially injurious to those with a

tendency to troubles of this nature. The diseases which
have been mentioned in the etiology of these various complaints should be treated in such a way as to prevent their
serving as a possible cause of infection of the liver. If
any of these acute forms of inflammation do develop, rest
of both body and digestive organs should be enjoined. In
the early stages, cold applications may be of service in
reducing congestion, but later if there is quite severe pain
hot compresses will be of greater service. Care should be
exercised in the use of cathartics which may have an irritating effect upon the organ, both from the standpoint
of prophylaxis and especially after the trouble has arisen.
The remedies which have an influence on inflammatory
processes elsewhere will be of material benefit, and in addition remedies which act especially upon the liver may
be of service if indications point to thir use.

Belladonna 3x:—Extreme sensitiveness to touch; there
is throbbing pain in some cases, although this remedy may
be useful without such symptom, especially where there
are indications that pus may form if relief be not secured.
There are flushed face, high temperature, and the general
sthenic condition of this remedy.

Bryonia 3x:—Sharp, stitching pains, which are greatly
aggravated by motion. The skin is more dusky than in
the belladonna patient; much thirst, dry, white tongue;
irritability is especially marked upon trying to move,
as may be desired for purpose of examination.

Rhus toxicodendron 3x:—Greater prostration than in
the preceding remedies. Although the patient seems weak,
there is inclination to move and seek an easier position.
Patient may be verging on typhoid symptoms, or they may
be fully developed.

China 2x :—If chill, fever and sweat occur in regular and distinct order. There is considerable prostration, much thirst and headache. Particularly indicated in cases secondary to malaria. Possibly when existing with malaria, stronger doses may be of greater service, even quinia sulphate in material doses. On the other hand there is no doubt if quinia is used in too large doses, or for too protracted a period it may have an influence in inducing an inflammatory condition in the liver.

Chelidonium 3x :—With feeling of a fulness in the liver, with enlargement that can be detected by physical examination. There is the characteristic sharp, lancinating pain under the right shoulder blade.

Podophyllum 6x :—There is pain especially marked in some one spot. A bitter taste and bilious symptoms. Some icterus, especially of the conjunctivæ. May be an associated enteritis with diarrhœa that is changeable in color and general appearance.

Leptandra 3x :—Likely to be some icterus. Soreness in the head and eye-balls. The especially characteristic symptom is the presence of black fetid stools.

Nux vomica 3x :—Due to excessive eating and the use of intoxicating liquors. Shooting pains through the liver, which is very sensitive to pressure. The patient feels weak and prostrated and is short of breath, especially after eating and upon exertion. There is constipation.

Mercurius solubilis 3x :—Useful in the interstitial and parenchymatous forms, but especially indicated where pus formation is threatened. If there is dysentery the mercurius corrosivus will probably be of greater use both for the intestinal trouble and also for the purpose of remedying a threatened abscess of the liver. With these remedies there is apt to be great tendency to sweat, especially at night, with resulting prostration but no particular effect in relieving the fever or other symptoms. A large flabbly tongue and possibly salivation.

Hepar sulphur, lachesis and *arsenic* may be useful if pus has formed or is forming, but if present to any extent the case at once becomes surgical. If there is any possibility of so doing it should be evacuated and drained.

CHAPTER VI.

CIRRHOSIS OF THE LIVER.

This disease is of two kinds:

1.—Atrophic.

2.—Hypertrophic.

Atrophic cirrhosis of the liver is the name given to a chronic inflammation involving especially the interstitial tissue, and resulting in its excessive development. The parenchymatous or cellular elements of the organ also are affected, especially in the later stages, being compressed by the fibrous elements to such an extent that they may undergo some form of degeneration.

Etiology:—The chief etiological factor in the causation of atrophic cirrhosis of the liver is a continued indulgence in alcoholic liquors. However, some idiosyncrasy or other element must be present, because if this were not so it would seem that it would be more frequently present than is the case. The distilled liquors are more apt to cause the condition than are the wines and beers. Alcohol is also more apt to cause this trouble when taken daily, even in small amounts, than when taken at irregular intervals in much larger quantities. It is also more apt to be injurious when taken into an empty stomach than when taken after eating. Those who take a so-called "eye opener" in the morning before breakfast seem especially prone to cirrhosis of the liver.

Other causes may produce the disease, in fact cases have been reported where it was congenital. At such times, it is generally, though not always in the off-spring of parents who were addicted to intoxicants, or were syphilitic. Adults sometimes suffer from this disease as a result of syphilis, but this does not occur as often as it does in children who have a syphilitic heredity. Malaria may act as a causative agent, and it has been claimed that certain of the infectious diseases may have a tendency to start the trouble. It is probable though, that when it has followed infectious disease, it was in the cases of those who had been addicted to the use of liquor, even if only in small amounts, provided it was taken with daily regularity. In some rare cases, none of the above causes have seemed to exert any influence in its production, and it has been suggested that the absorption of bacterial toxins from the intestine into the liver, might be responsible.

Pathology:—The changes occur very slowly and in most cases probably begin long before the existence of the disease is suspected. The earlier changes can be studied only in patients who die from some other disease, and are of such a nature that they can be seen only with the microscope. The first to make their appearance are found in the region of distribution of the portal veins and consist in an increase of the interlobular connective tissue. It becomes more fibrous than normal and also contains some elastic tissue, which at first is between the lobules, but later penetrates into their substance. Numerous blood vessels are found in the new tissue, all of them belonging to the hepatic artery instead of to the portal vein. In fact, branches of the portal vein are so constricted by the new fibrous tissue, that less than the normal amount of blood can reach the lobules from this source. As a result, and also because of compression of the hepatic cells by the encompassing new fibrous and elastic tissue, the parenchyma undergoes either granular or fatty degeneration, and then atrophies. In this later stage the liver is shrunken, and on cross section seems hard and the cut surface is rough and granular, each of the granules being a constricted lobule. For a short time, in the earlier stage, it is probable that if the liver was examined it would be found to be larger than normal. This condition is because the contracting fibres prevent the return flow of blood from the liver by the venous circulation, and this results in a passive hyperæmia.

Symptomatology:—In the early stages of hepatic cirrhosis symptoms are not prominent. If any are present they are apt to be only those indicating dyspepsia, and quite similar to symptoms present in those who use spirituous liquors, but who have not developed cirrhosis of the liver. After a variable length of time, possibly some years after the process has begun, symptoms of a more decided nature make their appearance, though even at this time they may not be sufficiently characteristic to warrant an undoubted diagnosis. When fully developed the symptoms of this disease may be considered in three divisions:

1.—Those of the liver itself.

2.—Those of other organs.

3.—Constitutional symptoms.

There is usually an increased sensitiveness in the hepatic region. In some cases there may even be pain, either of a dull, aching character or sharp and lancinating. This pain is apt to be due more to an associated peri-hepatitis

than to the atrophic process. Objectively in the early
stage there is an increased size in the area of hepatic dullness, which may be determined by palpation and percussion. It is known that later the liver shrinks up into the
cupola of the diaphragm, but this is more difficult to
demonstrate by physical methods than is the preceding
hypertrophy. This difficulty may be due partly to the associated ascites, to intestinal tympanitis and to emphysema of the lungs, any of these conditions obscuring the
percussion note of a normal liver. On the other hand, the
organ may be so adherent to the parieties with which it
is in contact, that its surface can not contract sufficiently
to destroy the hepatic dullness. If none of these conditions are present, it is usually possible to detect a considerable decrease in the size of the liver after the process
has existed for a sufficient length of time.

The conditions existing in other organs may be due to
the alcoholism, malaria or syphilis acting primarily, or
they may be due to the cirrhotic process independent of
these etiological agents. If due to the cirrhosis, such
changes are largely the effects produced on the portal circulation. The hardening liver compresses the terminals
of the portal vein, and as a result there is a stasis extending to all the tributaries which go to make up the portal
system. Thus the walls of the stomach suffer a passive
congestion because of obstruction to the gastric and pyloric veins. The spleen is swollen and indurated because
of obstruction to the veins leading from this organ. There
are apt to be hæmorrhoids because the rectum is not normally drained by the inferior mesenteric vein. Of especial importance is a stasis in the branches which go to
make up the mesenteric veins. These vessels, draining as
they do from the intestine and peritoneum, act imperfectly

in this condition and as a result there is an exudate from these surfaces which constitutes the condition called ascites. This, in most cases, is a symptom of the later stages, not being present until the cirrhotic process has made considerable progress. When it does arise, it is one of the most prominent symptoms of the disease. A limited amount of ascites may cause no trouble, and in many cases probably exists for some time before it is detected, especially in obese patients. The ascitic fluid is straw colored, of a specific gravity of from 1012 to 1014 and contains about 1% of albumen. Sometimes it is hæmorrhagic or bile stained. When portal stasis becomes marked, the collateral veins become dilated. In this manner the inferior œsophageal veins may become so enlarged that they rupture, giving rise perhaps to hæmatemesis. The venous connections between the liver and diaphragm become enlarged. The caput medusæ is a name given to an enlargement of the abdominal veins about the umbilicus, which is sometimes present. If the ascites is pronounced, the diaphragm and the heart are crowded upward and respiration and the systemic circulation are thus affected. Partly because of this interference with the action of the heart, and also to some extent because of the pressure of the ascites on the veins leading from the lower extremities, there may be œdema of the feet and legs. The kidneys are to some extent compressed, and this together with the impeded absorption of fluid by the intestinal mucous membrane results in a scanty secretion of urine.

Constitutionally, the patient's health and nutrition are much impaired. He becomes weak, and his muscles are flabby. The complexion is sallow and occasionally is icteric, though jaundice is not a marked symptom. In the later stages he becomes emaciated, although this may be more real than apparent, because of the œdema and ascites. The weakness and emaciation are due partly to poor absorption in the intestine and partly to interference with metabolism as a result of destruction of liver cells. Due to the imperfect metabolism, there is a decreased excretion of urea and an increase of ammonia in the urine. In a few cases there is sugar in the urine. Hæmorrhages may be present manifesting themselves in the nasal, pulmonary and urinary passages or they may appear as petechiæ in the skin, retina, pleura or peritoneum. Slight fever with rapid and weakened pulse may be present. Nephritis, meningitis, myocarditis, arterio-sclerosis and splenic cirrhosis may all be present, possibly caused by the same things which caused the hepatic cirrhosis, or possibly secondary to this disease. The peritoneum often becomes chronically inflamed, and it is said that tuberculosis of this membrane is quite a frequent complication. In the latest stages the liver sometimes undergoes fatty or amyloid degeneration and abscess or carcinoma may develop within its substance.   .

Diagnosis:—In the earlier stage a diagnosis is often quite difficult. If the patient has indulged in alcoholic drinks for a long period, it is an argument in favor of cirrhosis, although the disease may arise without such a history, and, of course, other diseases of the liver may occur in chronic alcoholics. The very slow development of the diseased picture shown above indicates cirrhosis. Many of the symptoms are found in other troubles, but they are apt to come on more rapidly at such times. Physical examination of the liver in the earlier stages will generally show that the organ is somewhat enlarged, later that it is atrophied, except when some of the conditions mentioned in the symptomatology are present and prevent a shrinking of its surface. A diagnosis of the ascites may usually be made by eliciting a percussion wave, although ascites may be due to other conditions than cirrhosis of the liver. This matter will be considered more fully in studying the diseases of the peritoneum. Enlargement of the venules of the surface of the abdomen, around the umbilicus, or in other regions, will in most cases indicate the disease under consideration.

Prognosis:—The final outcome of cirrhosis of the liver is always death. However, the process is so slow that some intercurrent disease is quite apt to develop and close the scene. When death has occurred from another disease with no suspicion of this trouble being present, we frequently find, at autopsy, evidence of a beginning cirrhosis of the liver. If the disease is allowed to progress to its termination, many years generally lapse before the end. However when it has reached a stage where marked symptoms are present it advances more rapidly, and a fatal termination may be expected within a comparatively short time. It is in the earlier period, before very decided symptoms have arisen that slow progress is to be expected. Once in a while a case will seemingly recover, but at such times it is probable that a mistake was made in the diagnosis, although possibly when due to syphilis or something else besides alcoholism, improvement or entire recovery may be effected.

Treatment:—Of chief importance is a cessation of the alcoholic habit. Spices, coffee and other irritating articles of diet should also be eliminated. It is better to limit to a considerable extent the starches and sugars, and somewhat, the fats. A milk diet for a long time is often of benefit, and if the symptoms are marked, even more relief may be obtained by the employment of skimmed milk. If there is great craving for the customary stimulants, koumiss may be judiciously used with some benefit. Constipation with its attendant absorption of toxins should be combated by means other than irritating laxatives. Enemata will in most cases be most satisfactory for this purpose.

Nux vomica 3x:—To counteract the bad effects of alcohol, this remedy has a well earned reputation, and for that reason is often beneficial in this complaint. Of course it has no effect in removing the excess of connective tissue developed, but for relief of many of the subjective symptoms it will be useful. There are the customary nervous irritability, slight icterus, coated tongue, belching of gas and sour fluids, constipation, hæmorrhoids and general exhaustion.

China 3x:—Where there is a history of malaria, with possibly a periodicity of the symptoms, and considerable flatulence, weakness and enlargement of the liver, this remedy will be useful. If the malaria has been quite recent, quinine in moderate sized material doses may have a better influence.

Iodide of potash:—This is the principal remedy if there is a history of syphilis, and even when there is not such a history it will sometimes be of value. It should generally be given in doses of from five to fifteen grains.

Mercurius:—In syphilitic cases, in material doses. It is also useful in attenuation for dyspeptic and other symptoms which may be found in cases not due to syphilis. At such times there will be some sensitiveness in the region of the liver, aggravated by lying on the right side. There is apt to be slight icterus, the characteristic tongue. The symptoms will often be aggravated at night.

Phosphorus 6x:—In its provings, this remedy gives rise to both pathology and symptoms quite similar to cirrhosis of the liver, so it seemingly should be useful in its treatment. When particularly indicated it will be of use, but because of its especial ability to produce a similar pathology, it has been used in cases that did not present an especially similar group of other symptoms, and as it did not prove of value it has fallen into disrepute. There is more tenderness than in many of the remedies, especially upon pressure and during the hypertrophic stage. Great weakness and prostration, particularly of a nervous character. A feeling of fulness in the epigastrium, often with nausea especially shortly after drinking cold water. Quite a tendency to hæmorrhages in various parts of the body, the blood being watery and not easy to coagulate. In the late stages when there is a tendency to fatty degeneration.

Aurum muriaticum 2x:—This is a favorite remedy with many for cirrhotic processes in any organ. There should be the mental symptoms of despondency with inclination to commit suicide. Exceedingly peevish; becomes vehement upon contradiction. There may be immoderate appetite, and yet the stomach feels qualmish. In the hepatic region there is a burning sensation or a cutting pain.

For the ascites, abdominal paracentesis is generally most practicable. Of course it is not curative, and as a rule if it is once commenced it has to be continued at frequent intervals. But it gives great relief for a time, and in some cases when combined with other treatment will improve the abdominal circulation so that the patient will feel better for quite awhile, and the ascites may be kept from returning to so great an extent. The fluid may also be drained away be strong cathartics, especially elaterium 1/10 to ⅛ grain doses, or by such diuretics as the digitalis infusion. These methods however are more prostrating than the aspirator, and not as satisfactory.

In recent years operative measures have been employed in treating cirrhosis of the liver. Scarifying its surface has been done, so as to cause adhesions to the abdominal parieties and thus improve its collateral circulation. This also causes adhesions with the omentum. Varying reports have been made as to the success of such methods, but at present they do not seem to have been very satisfactory, and such operations are not advised by the majority of operators.

CHAPTER VII.

HYPERTROPHIC CIRRHOSIS.

Definition:—A condition where the connective tissue of the liver is increased in amount but does not result in a destruction or diminution of the parenchymatous tissue, as is the case in atrophic cirrhosis.

Etiology:—It is a much more rare condition than the atrophic variety, and its existence was not recognized until a few years ago. It has been most carefully studied by the French physicians, and it is thought to occur more frequently in that country than elsewhere. Young men from 20 to 30 years of age seem to be most susceptible to the disease, although it has also been found in children. The exciting cause is unknown. It has been claimed by some that alcohol has an effect in causing it, others have denied such an etiology. Certain bacteria have been found which were thought by their discoverers to have produced the trouble, but their claims have not been substantiated by other investigators. Syphilis and malaria seem to have no influence in its production.

Pathology:—The chief change is an increase in the amount of connective tissue separating the lobules. This increase may become enormous so that the liver causes the right costal arch to bulge outward, and it may extend downward to the crest of the ilium. The organ retains its normal shape in most cases, though exceptionally the left lobe may become somewhat irregular in form. The connective tissue consists of fine fibrils, between which are many nests of young cells and also some elastic tissue. The interlobular bile passages located in this new connective tissue become two or three times their normal thickness, and are very tortuous. Their lumen may remain patulous or become obstructed by desquamated epithelium or flakes of pigment. The blood vessels of both the portal system and the hepatic artery remain totally unchanged. The same may be said of the liver cells, at least until the fatal termination approaches, at which time a fatty degeneration of the parenchyma may take place.

Symptomatology:—In the beginning, there are simply attacks of a dyspeptic nature. These outbreaks occur at intervals of several months, or even longer, and are accompanied by pronounced icterus and painful enlargement of the liver. Their severity usually increases as does also their frequency, and after a few attacks the hepatic enlargement remains during the intervals. There is loss of appetite, flatulence, nausea, vomiting, epigastric distress and probably fever. In fact the general symptoms are almost identical with those occurring in catarrhal cholangitis. The skin may become lightly or heavily jaundiced, although there is always sufficient bile entering the intestine to keep the fæces well stained. The liver becomes so enlarged that palpation and percussion show it to occupy much more space than normal, and it is very sensitive to pressure. The spleen becomes much enlarged. There are apt to be hæmorrhages, as epistaxis, purpura, bleeding of the gums and of the intestines. As the case progresses, the attacks come closer together until at last there is no freedom. Toward the end, the appetite may increase, and sometimes bulimia exists. However eating seems to do no good, as malnutrition develops and the patient dies in the end from general exhaustion. Although death is the final outcome it does not take place for years, and during this time there may be protracted intervals when the patient feels comparatively well.

Diagnosis:—In the earlier stage the disease can not be diagnosed, as the attacks so closely resemble catarrhal cholangitis, but in time it may be seen that they are accompanied by an advancing enlargement of the liver, which is smooth and regular in form. There is also a persistent jaundice, which is not accompanied by a loss of color in the stools. There is enlarged spleen and there is no ascites.

Treatment:—In the beginning the treatment is chiefly that for gastric and intestinal catarrh and for congestion of the liver. A non-irritating diet without alcohol is indicated. The remedies may be selected from those mentioned under the above diseases, their indications being the same as in such troubles.

CHAPTER VIII.

DEGENERATIVE DISEASES OF THE LIVER.

Degenerative processes of the hepatic parenchyma may be of two kinds:

1.—Fatty.

2.—Amyloid.

Fatty changes in the liver may be in the form of either infiltration or degeneration. Fatty infiltration occurs to a limited extent even in normal livers, as the cells always contain small globules of oil. In people who are inclined to be obese this infiltration is still more prominently displayed. However, this process can hardly be considered pathological inasmuch as symptoms never result.

Fatty degeneration, which is a change of the protoplasm of the hepatic cells to fat, is a comparatively rare condition and occurs in the following ways:

1.—As a part of general obesity in which fatty infiltration takes place first, while later the degenerative process is also initiated.

2.—In cases where for some reason oxidation in the body is lowered. This is seen in anæmia, phthisis and other diseases of this type.

3.—Where for some reason an increased demand for oxygen is made upon the tissues of the body and especially of the liver. This chiefly applies to those who imbibe too freely of alcohol.

4.—Some poisons possess the power of so damaging the protoplasm that it undergoes fatty degeneration. Phosphorus is the principal one which acts in this manner.

Symptomatology:—As important an organ as is the liver, it seems peculiar that such great changes can take place in its protoplasm without producing more prominent symptoms. The patient generally suffers from the symptoms of the primary disease which caused the fatty liver, more noticeably than from those due to this condition. In fact, there are none of the characteristic signs such as jaundice, ascites or other symptoms which might be expected. If the patient is obese it may be difficult by physical methods to detect positively the changes which have occurred. If the abdominal walls are thin it may be found that the organ is enlarged, in some cases to a great extent. If in tuberculosis of the lungs or cachectic conditions this enlargement, which is soft, smooth and causes no pain, can be detected, the disease under consideration may generally be diagnosed.

Treatment:—Attention to the causative disease is of chief importance. For instance, if general obesity is marked an endeavor should be made to get rid of this tendency by the means generally employed. If phthisis or other disease interfering with oxidation in the body exists, radical treatment should be used for its improvement. Alcoholic or other habits calling for such an amount of oxygen in the body that the tissues must be called upon to help supply the demand, should be corrected, and if poisons such as phosphorus have gained access to the body, means should be employed to stimulate their elimination and to antidote their effects. When not caused by phosphorus this element seems in a pathological way to be strictly homœopathic to the condition, and for this reason has been employed in attenuated form in its treatment. If others than the pathological symptoms are present in a given case it will probably be of value, but experience with it shows that it does not possess sufficient power as a rule to have very much effect in delaying the process, and certainly none in causing the fat to change back into the normal, healthy protoplasm of hepatic tissue.

The exact nature of the change which takes place in the liver and is called amyloid, waxy or lardaceous degeneration, is not thoroughly understood. It is found in patients who have had some long, serious disease, frequently though it need not always be of a suppurative nature, and who have developed a decided cachexia. Tuberculosis of the lungs or bones is most often the primary condition. Next to this comes syphilis, and in rare cases it is found in rickets and after severe attacks of some of the infectious fevers.

Pathology:—The process begins in the center of the lobules, first attacking the capillary blood vessels. Later, the vessels between the lobules undergo the same change, and lastly, the connective tissue. The hepatic cells usually escape, although in some cases which have continued for some time and become extremely severe, some degeneration may take place in the cells. The amyloid substance is semi-translucent, appears anæmic and is very solid and firm in consistency. The organ as a whole in most cases increases very markedly in size, sometimes assuming gigantic proportions. In exceptional cases instead of becoming enlarged, it undergoes atrophy.

Symptomatology:—Like fatty degeneration, this process gives rise to no definite symptoms. Jaundice, ascites and dyspeptic symptoms are absent, or if present seem to be entirely independent of this affection. The secretion of bile goes on the same as in the normal liver, although occasionally the stools become light colored.

Diagnosis:—This can generally be made quite easily. The disease exists only in those who have long been afflicted with the affections mentioned in the etiology, and if in such cases the liver on physical examination is found to be greatly enlarged, with a hard smooth surface, with edges prominent and easily felt, amyloid degeneration is present.

Treatment:—This consists only in trying to remedy the original disease. Treatment for this process itself is unavailing.

CHAPTER IX.
TUMORS OF THE LIVER.

The new growths which develop in the liver may be either cystic or solid. Of the cystic growths, the echino-cocci may be mentioned, but as they are extremely rare in this country and have already been mentioned when considering the subject of parasites, they will be given no space at this time. Other forms of cysts which are sometimes found in this organ may be designated as simple and multiple.

Simple cysts are very rare and are probably always due to some malformation. The most notable ones which have been described were due to such abnormal conditions as accessory liver, accessory gall bladder and fistulous communications with the suspensory ligament, with mucous glands on the liver surface and with isolated bile passages not communicating with the main bile duct.

Multiple cysts are generally associated with an abnormal condition of the bile passages, as for instance when they do not terminate in the liver substance, but end blindly in the region of the suspensory ligament. Such abnormality may be congenital or may be secondary to other pathological processes, especially cirrhosis of the liver.

Pathology:—The cysts hold an albuminous fluid containing mucin, epithelium, leucocytes, red corpuscles and cholesterin. Bile pigment is generally absent. The color of the fluid may be watery, yellowish or brown. They vary in size from an almost microscopic point to a foot in diameter.

Symptomatology:—These cysts may give rise to no symptoms unless they are large enough to cause compression of the surrounding liver substance. At such times they cause ascites, possibly swelling of the spleen, and congestive catarrh of the stomach and intestine. The kidneys may also be affected in a similar manner.

Diagnosis:—The only positive way to determine that an hepatic enlargement is cystic in nature, is to obtain some of the fluid by aspiration.

Treatment:—Unless giving rise to active symptoms no treatment is advisable. If, on account of their size they are affecting the health, the only method of obtaining relief from their presence is by aspiration or drainage.

Solid tumors of the liver may be either benign or malignant. The benign growths are extremely rare; in fact they may be considered as medical curiosities. Fibromata and angiomata have been reported. They give rise to no characteristic symptoms, and can be diagnosed only at operation or at autopsy. Because of these reasons and also because of their rarity no further mention will be made of them.

Of malignant neoplasms, sarcomata may be mentioned only to say that they are also extremely rare. Their presence as primary growths has been denied, although they are sometimes found in the liver as a result of metastasis from other organs. Recently however a very few have been reported as occurring primarily.

Carcinoma of the liver occurs more frequently than any other form of tumor of this organ. It may be either secondary to a cancer originating in some other organ or it may be primary. When the former, its presence here may be due to extension by contiguity from either the stomach, duodenum, colon, pancreas or gall bladder. When occurring through metastasis, it may come from almost any other organ, but especially from those already mentioned and also from the breast, mediastinum, rectum or uterus.

Pathology :—Carcinomatous growths of the liver may assume any one of three different anatomical types:

1.—Nodulated cancer.

2.—Cirrhotic cancer.

3.—Massive cancer.

The nodular type is the one generally found in secondary growths, and in the primary ones is more frequent than either of the other varieties. The nodules may be quite numerous and vary from the size of a pin-head to that of an orange. Generally one of the large ones is apparently the starting point of the growth, and the other ones are grouped around this chief nodule. When primary, it rarely reaches a very large size. When secondary, as a result of metastasis from some other organ, it sometimes reaches gigantic proportions.

In the cirrhotic cancer there seems to be some relationship between the carcinoma and cirrhosis of the liver. It is not known positively which affection is primary or acts etiologically. This form is also somewhat nodular in character, though not to the extent of the preceding variety. In addition to the increase of the epithelial elements typical of cancer, there is also an increased development of the connective tissue as seen in cirrhosis. In some cases this increase is but slight, at other times it is very large. The size of the liver depends to a large extent upon the quantity of the connective tissue. If there is much of this, the viscus may become atrophied, while if the increase in epithelial elements predominates, it may retain its normal size, or even become enlarged.

The massive cancer is most rare. It is always primary and most often develops in the right lobe. It grows rapidly, it is solitary, its edges are sharply defined, and it is usually globular in shape. The surface of the liver may remain smooth, or have but few and small prominences. The growth is apt to start in the middle of the lobe and be surrounded by healthy liver substance. There is no increase in the connective tissue. By continuity the growth may in time extend to the gall bladder, right kidney or peritoneum. Metastases from the growth are rare except possibly to the lymphatics situated in the hilus of the organ.

Symptomatology:—Many times the symptoms which first attract attention in cancer of the liver are of a general nature. There will be a gradual loss of flesh and strength. Coming a little later will be found digestive disturbances such as anorexia, nausea and vomiting. In cases of the so-called massive cancer there will be considerable enlargement of the organ which is perceptible by inspection, palpation and percussion. To a lesser extent there is also enlargement in the majority of cases of the nodular variety, while in a few of this kind and all of the cirrhotic cancer type the liver will be smaller than normal. In the nodular and cirrhotic forms, the surface of the organ will feel irregular upon palpation and generally be somewhat tender to touch. The massive cancer will be smooth. In most cases there is some pain, or at least a feeling of uneasiness in the hepatic region, although there are some which assume very large proportions and yet give rise to no local distress. Jaundice is present in about half of the cases, and is generally moderate in extent, unless the growth is so located that the common duct is pressed upon, when there is marked jaundice. Ascites is not often present except in the cirrhotic variety, when the portal vein is compressed, or when there is extension to

the peritoneum. When the growth has advanced to a considerable degree, there is often fever, running generally
from 100° to 102°, mostly continuous, but sometimes intermittent and with a wider variation. This latter condition is more apt to be present if suppuration develops.
Cachexia and anæmia are marked. Resulting from the
anæmia there is often œdema in various parts of the body,
especially the lower extremities. It is impossible from the
symptoms to determine whether the cancer of the liver is
primary or secondary, unless the original growth can be
discovered in some other part, as the breast, stomach, rectum or elsewhere.

Diagnosis:—This comprises a determination both as to
whether a new growth is of the liver, or whether it is of
the gall bladder, stomach, duodenum, hepatic flexure of
the colon, pancreas or right kidney. And, if determined
to be of the liver, whether it is cancer, cyst, fatty or amyloid liver or cirrhosis.

In cancer of the gall bladder there is generally a history of gall stones; jaundice is more often present, appears earlier and is more intense; the tumor is shaped
more like a gall bladder and is located at that point. It
may be difficult to determine cancer of the left lobe from
the same disease in the stomach, but in the latter there is
apt to be more vomiting and more severe pain. A line
of tympanitis may be defined between the tumor and the
right lobe of the liver and finally examination of the
stomach contents will show their peculiar characteristics.
The same points with the exception of examination of the
stomach contents will apply in differentiating between
cancer of the liver and of the duodenum or colon. Cancer
of the pancreas may generally be distinguished by examination of the stools, or by distending the stomach with

air. If it is a growth of the pancreas, the stomach will be anterior to the growth, if of the liver it will be posterior.

If the growth is determined to be in the liver, it may be differentiated from fatty or amyloid degeneration by the history, the jaundice, the more rapid growth, the greater cachexia and the usually nodulated surface. Some cases of amyloid degeneration with syphilitic gummata may be nodular, but they will generally clear up under syphilitic treatment. Cysts, especially those due to the echinococcus, may resemble cancer, but their nodules are usually softer to the touch. If we are unable to determine positively, aspiration may be carefully performed in an endeavour to find cystic contents. It may be impossible at first to diagnose between cancer and hypertrophic cirrhosis. The latter trouble however, lacks the severe cachexia and the nodular surface, and has less pain. Cirrhotic cancer and simple cirrhosis may be difficult to differentiate, and it may be necessary to wait until the more rapid decline shows it to be cancer.

Prognosis:—Death follows in all cases, usually in less than eighteen months, more often in less than a year.

Treatment:—Medical treatment is only palliative, endeavoring to keep up the nutrition and to relieve pain and suffering. Attempts have been made to give relief by operation, and if diagnosed early enough possibly success may be attained in some cases.

Part VI.—Diseases of the Pancreas.

CHAPTER I.

The inflammatory diseases of this organ may be classified as,—

1.—Acute hæmorrhagic pancreatitis.
2.—Suppurative pancreatitis.
3.—Chronic pancreatitis.

Because of the comparative inaccessibility of this organ, its affections have in the past been but little understood, and it has been thought its diseases were rare. Probably this is true, yet more recent investigations have tended to the idea that they were more frequent than had been believed, and that sometimes affections which have been diagnosed as gastric or other diseases, have in reality been located in the pancreas. If recovery ensued, the mistake would not be discovered. Yet careful and extensive pathological investigations have failed to find the various types of inflammatory diseases in any great number of autopsies. For instance in a series of 18,509 autopsies performed at the Vienna Krankenhaus reports showed only one case of acute hæmorrhagic pancreatitis, nine cases of the suppurative form and five cases of chronic pancreatitis. Therefore, as these lesions are so rare it does not seem advisable to give a great deal of space to their consideration.

ACUTE HÆMORRHAGIC PANCREATITIS.

Etiology:—In this form the inflammation and the hæmorrhage are so closely associated that it is impossible to determine which is primary, or in other words which is cause and which is effect. It occurs more frequently in adult males, probably because the use of alcohol in excessive amounts seems to be an etiological factor. In women it occasionally exists in relation to pregnancy and parturition. It may also take place in connection with gall stone colic. It has been found by experiment on dogs, that a similar pathological condition may be produced by blocking the bile duct in such a manner that the bile is allowed to regurgitate into the pancreas. Therefore by inference it is assumed that the same thing may occur in the human being, as a result of a similar blockade by a gall stone.

Pathology :—At autopsy, the pancreas is found considerably enlarged with blood between the lobules. The blood may be fluid or clotted, and in the substance of the lobules themselves there may be a bloody serum causing a condition of œdema. The pancreatic cells undergo necrosis, and this process also extends to other tissues outside of this organ. For instance necrotic spots of an ivory color and which may be mistaken for tubercles are found distributed throughout the abdominal cavity, especially in the mesentery and omentum.

Symptomatology :—An attack is ushered in by the sudden appearance of extreme pain. The swelling of the pancreas causes an involvement of the cœliac plexus, and it is supposed that pain is made more agonizing by this fact. There is nausea, vomiting, great prostration, rapid pulse, dyspnœa and rapid loss of strength. In some cases there is a chill, possibly with subnormal temperature as a result of shock, and fever may follow. The bowels are extremely constipated, in most cases there seeming to be complete intestinal obstruction. Within a short time the abdomen becomes swollen, and a circumscribed enlargement may sometimes be palpated in the pancreatic region,

There is delirium, many times merging into coma. Death has usually taken place within four days at most, sometimes even earlier.

Diagnosis:—The cases so far reported have generally been mistaken for either perforative peritonitis or acute intestinal obstruction. To make an absolute differentiation seems impossible, and as these other conditions are so much more common, the same mistakes will probably continue, to be discovered only at autopsy or at operation. Fitz has said that, "acute pancreatitis may be suspected when a previously healthy person or a sufferer from occasional attacks of indigestion is suddenly seized with a violent pain in the epigastrium followed by vomiting and collapse, and in the course of twenty-four hours by a circumscribed epigastric swelling, tympanitic or resistant, with slight elevation of temperature. Circumscribed tenderness in the course of the pancreas and tender spots throughout the abdomen are valuable diagnostic signs."

SUPPURATIVE PANCREATITIS.

Etiology:—This form may evidently be either primary or secondary. In the primary form the infection in most cases probably extends up the excretory duct from the intestine in the same manner that it does in causing infection of the bile tract by extending up the common bile duct. In fact, considering the frequency of the latter condition, it seems peculiar that infection of the pancreas does not occur oftener than it does. Another method by which the infecting bacteria may gain entrance, is by penetrating from other areas in the neighborhood, as for instance from an ulcer of the stomach. It has been considered that predisposing causes are alcoholism, suppression of menstruation, pregnancy and the use of mercury. However, abscess of the pancreas is so rare that not sufficient study has been possible to enable us to arrive at positive conclusions in regard to the matter.

Secondary or metastatic abscesses may occur in the pancreas as a result of the bacteria being carried to the organ from other places. Pyæmia, puerperal fever, parotitis and probably primary abscess in almost any part of the body may be originating factors.

Pathology :—The suppuration may exist either as a single large abscess or as multiple small foci. As in the acute hæmorrhagic form, so-called fat necrosis is apt to be present not only in the organ itself but also in the surrounding parts. Necrosis or gangrene of the entire pancreas or a large part of it may also take place as a termination in either of these diseases. When this happens the gangrene may be of either the dry or the moist type.

Symptomatology :—Suppurative pancreatitis generally begins suddenly. At first there is severe pain in this region, radiating over the entire abdomen, although cases have been reported in which there were no pains. There is marked tenderness, eructations, nausea and often vomiting. Fever is generally present, irregular and often alternating with chills. At first there may be either constipation or diarrhœa but after the first twenty-four hours there is a profuse diarrhœa. Blood and fetid smelling pus may be in the stools, and the presence of large quantities of fat and albumen shows the effects of imperfect intestinal digestion. The epigastric region becomes distended and tympanitic, sometimes presenting a tumor or at least appearing resistant. The other organs of the abdomen may become affected, especially the liver and spleen, although cases have been reported where they did not seem to be changed to any extent.

Diagnosis:—The majority of cases reported were not diagnosed until either operation or autopsy. The symptoms mentioned are so much more apt to occur in other troubles that it seldom seems justifiable to make a diagnosis of pancreatic abscess from them alone. However, if the symptoms mentioned above are present, and a tumor or resistance can be made out which is located behind the omental bursa, the presence of this affection may be considered.

CHRONIC PANCREATITIS.

Etiology:—This condition probably exists, at least in mild form, more frequently than has been realized in the past. In nearly all cases it is secondary to some kind of obstruction to the duct of Wirsung. The obstructive agent may be gall stones lodged in the common bile duct, pancreatic calculi or tumors of some adjoining organ. Operative measures upon the bile tract quite often show that the pancreas has undergone one of the two forms of sclerotic changes mentioned below. It is not thoroughly understood how gall stones or bile tract disease produce the condition. It was formerly thought that it was by the obstruction alone, this allowing a blocking or regurgitation of pancreatic juice. Others have advanced the idea that certain lymphatics which have their origin in the gall bladder and bile ducts and terminate in the pancreas, especially in its head, act as agents of conveyance of the necessary infection.

Pathology:—There are two varieties of pathology found in chronic pancreatitis, which compare very closely to the atrophic and hypertrophic forms of cirrhosis of the liver. They may be called the interlobular and the interacinar. In the interlobular form, there is an increase of the fibrous tissue which at first is confined to the spaces between the lobules. Later it creeps in from the periphery toward the center and finally the Islands of Langerhans are considerably involved. Owing to the large increase in the fibrous tissue, the organ appears more lobulated than normal and becomes considerably enlarged.

In the interacinar type there is formation of a net-work of fibrous tissue within the lobules themselves. The Islands of Langerhans thus become involved at a very early stage. Between the lobules there is but slight change. As a result the organ does not become nodular as in the other form, and to the touch appears smooth and soft.

Chronic pancreatitis may affect the entire gland or a part of it only. When the latter, the head is much more frequently diseased than the body or tail. In the case of the interlobular form affecting the head there is such a hardening and enlargement at the point where the common bile duct passes either close to the organ, or, as frequently happens, through a canal penetrating the head, that more or less obstruction is offered to the flow of bile. In such a case if a gall stone attempts to pass through the duct it is much more apt to become lodged, giving rise to jaundice and other serious symptoms. In operating at such times to remove the gall stone the head of the pancreas has sometimes appeared so enlarged and nodular that a diagnosis of cancer has been made, which later developments have shown to be a mistake.

Symptomatology :—The symptoms of chronic pancreatitis are mostly of a digestive nature. There is loss of appetite, especially for meats and fats. There may or may not be nausea and vomiting. A feeling of pressure is quite common together with flatulence, meteorism and colicky pains. There may be jaundice which is extremely persistent, and probably due to the hardening about the common bile duct interfering with the free passage of the bile. The particular symptoms directing attention especially to the pancreas are found in the altered conditions of the fæces and sometimes the urine. The stools are very bulky and frequent because food has been so imperfectly digested that absorption could not take place. They are paler than normal partly because of the large amount of undigested fat contained, a condition frequently met and called steatorrhœa, but more especially because of the absence of an insoluble pigment which is present in normal stools, as a result of the action of the pancreatic juice upon some of the coloring matters of the bile.

Diagnosis:—If the gland is diseased in the larger part of its area, there may usually be found in the stools under the microscope an increased number of striated muscle fibres. This condition is called azotorrhœa. In some cases the presence of fat may be determined by the greasy appearance of the stool to the naked eye, but a more exact method is by the test mentioned in the chapter treating of the examination of the fæces. To prove that steatorrhœa is due to pancreatic disease, a preparation of pancreatic extract may be administered, when there will be a considerable decrease in its amount. Such a test, as also examining the stools for an excess of mucus due to an enteritis, should be employed for the reason that in the latter disease the stools may contain both fat and albumen in excess, not because they have not been properly acted upon by the pancreatic juice but because the intestine was unable to absorb them. The possibility of cancer of the pancreas instead of inflammation must also be considered. One method of differentiating is by testing the stools for stercobilin. Cancer of the head of the pancreas preventing the passage of bile, obliterates the stercobilin from the fæces. In chronic pancreatitis although its amount is lessened, still sufficient is present to be detected.

The urine may be changed in inflammation of the pancreas. If the process has involved the Islands of Langerhans there is present a glycosuria in most cases. As noted in the pathology, this condition arises early in the interacinar type and late in the interlobular. At present, the most definite sign of pancreatitis is thought to be the so-called Cammidge reaction of the urine. Its presence is said by some to be positive proof of the presence of this condition. Unfortunately, however, the technic of this test is difficult and requires more time than can generally be given except by laboratory specialists. For these reasons no attempt will be made to give it in detail at this point. Slight errors in its performance are said to invalidate all conclusions which may be drawn from its presence, but when positive it always indicates the disease under consideration. It may be found in cancer of the pancreas in about one fourth of the cases, but only when the cancer is associated with inflammation. To provide for this contingency it should generally be performed in conjunction with the test for stercobilin in the fæces and by means of both of them a differentiation between the two diseases may usually be made.

Treatment:—Inflammatory diseases of the pancreas are notably unsatisfactory to treat. The acute varieties, if diagnosed, may be treated surgically, attempting to drain in the case of suppuration and to remove blood clots in the acute hæmorrhagic. In the chronic form, due as it is frequently to obstruction of the duct of Wirsung, attempts may also be made to remove the obstruction by surgical means. Operations for gall stones have probably relieved many cases of this form of the disease. Medically the diet may need to be regulated according to well known methods to meet conditions found in the urine and stool. For instance, in glycosuria the carbohydrates will need to be reduced: in fatty diarrhœa the fats should be made to meet the capabilities of digestion. Remedies are also to be selected according to indications more appropriately studied under other heads. In fact the subject of pancreatic disease is so imperfectly understood that no very definite treatment has been outlined, except in the case of diabetes of pancreatic origin. The more direct dyspeptic symptoms and their treatment by remedies have been sufficiently studied in other chapters of this book.

CHAPTER II.

PANCREATIC CYSTS.

Fluid accumulations developing within or upon the pancreas are sometimes found. They are quite rare, the entire list so far reported, which have been proven to be of this nature, numbering but 134 cases.

Etiology:—Considered from the standpoint of etiology there are three different types of pancreatic cysts.

1.—Retention cysts.
2.—Proliferation cysts.
3.—Apoplectic cysts.

The retention cysts are caused by some form of obstruction to the excretory ducts. This may be of the duct of Wirsung, or it may be within the substance of the organ and affect some of the smaller branches of the duct of Wirsung. Although obstruction is the necessary cause, yet it has been claimed by some that this is not the only factor, for in experiment upon animals ligation of the duct will cause only slight dilatation back of the ligature, not to an extent to cause anything which could be called a cyst. For this reason it has been supposed that there must be some abnormal condition either of the gland itself or of its secretion, which prevents absorption of the pancreatic juice after having been once formed, as seems to occur in the case of the ligature experiments. Whatever else may be necessary is therefore unknown, but as regards the obstruction itself it may be caused in four different ways.

1·—Chronic pancreatitis may result in such a development of new interstitial tissue that the ducts are compressed to such an extent that excretion is delayed or even prevented entirely. This is supposed to be the most common cause.

2.—Neoplasms from the pancreas itself or more commonly from adjoining organs may be so situated that the duct of Wirsung is compressed.

3.—Calculi of the pancreas, formed in the same manner as biliary calculi and probably from the same causes, have been reported in a few cases, and one or two such reports have shown that such calculi may become lodged in a manner so as to prevent the pancreatic secretion reaching the intestine, with a resulting cyst.

4.—It is probably a fact that simple catarrhal processes of the pancreatic ducts may produce such a thickening of the mucous lining that sufficient obstruction is present to cause the formation of a cyst.

Proliferation cysts may be regarded as an expression of the formation of cysts in tumors, or as a cystic degeneration of the pancreas itself, similar to that found in other glands, as the kidneys, testicles or mammæ.

. Apoplectic cysts are due to hæmorrhage within the pancreatic tissue as a result of the rupture of a blood vessel.

This variety is extremely rare and its existence is denied by some writers.

Symptomatology :—There is nothing particularly characteristic about the symptoms which are present in this affection. At first there are generally dyspeptic symptoms with gradual loss of weight and strength. Finally considerable pain makes its appearance, although this is inconstant, possibly being present in quite severe form for a time, then it may disappear for a time. At first it is in the epigastrium and seems to come from the stomach. Later it may radiate to other parts of the abdomen, towards the loins or the sacrum. It may appear at intervals in the form of colic, possibly of such severity as to cause fainting; at such times it is thought to be due to pressure by the cyst upon the solar plexus.

Vomiting is present in some patients, usually taking place during an attack of the pain, though later in the course of the disease it may come after each meal. If the vomiting is very severe it may at last be in the form of a hæmatemesis. The bowels may be normal, constipated or diarrhœic. In some cases there have been either steatorrhœa or azotorrhœa. However, in the majority of cases in which mention was made as to the nature of the stools, the presence of both these conditions were denied. In a few of the cases, there has been sugar reported in the urine, although this does not seem to be a necessary accompaniment. There is sometimes more or less jaundice, which is probably caused by pressure of the cyst upon the ductus communis choledochus. Pressure upon the ureter of one or the other kidney has also been reported. Ascites and œdema of the lower extremities may be present because the growth interferes with the return flow in the veins of the abdomen.

The physical signs are of importance because it is from these that the diagnosis must usually be made. As a rule the abdomen is distended, the section and degree of distention depending upon the location and size of the tumor. According to the surface of the pancreas from which the cyst develops and the direction of its growth, depends the relationship of the mass to the surrounding organs, especially the stomach, colon and liver. In the greater number of cases it projects forward between the stomach and colon. At times it remains behind the stomach pushing it forward, with the colon beneath, and in other cases it develops behind the transverse colon, pushing it forward, and with the stomach above the tumor.

Diagnosis:—Reports have shown that these cysts have been mistaken for a number of other conditions, as for instance, ovarian cysts, echinococci of the liver, aortic aneurysms, omental tumors, cysts of the peritoneum, of the mesentery, of the suprarenal gland, of the kidney, of the spleen, of the abdominal wall and for perinephritic abscess. Absolute differential points cannot be given between many of these conditions, and a positive diagnosis of this disease is in many cases very difficult. Determination of its location as regards the stomach, transverse colon and mesentery are of considerable value. Pancreatic cysts are strictly immovable, either upon respiration or by manipulation. Exploratory puncture to obtain some of the contents for examination has been practiced, but is not free from danger. If a specimen is obtained it may be examined as to the presence of the ferments. Those which act upon starch, fats and albumen should all be present, but the one which digests albumen is considered of chief importance. A fat emulsifying product is sometimes found in the contents of cysts of other organs.

Prognosis:—These cysts last for a long time, one case being reported where a growth which at forty-seven years of age was proven by operation to be of this nature, had been present since childhood. In other cases, they will appear suddenly and at once seem to affect the health very seriously or even be fatal. Cases have been reported where they had ruptured into the stomach or transverse colon causing sudden hæmorrhage, and possibly resulting in a permanent fistula which continued to eliminate pancreatic secretion.

Treatment:—Medical treatment is evidently of no avail in this disease. In recent years operative measures have been employed with considerable success. Of the 134 cases so far reported, the literature of which is available, 101 cases were operated upon, with 81 recoveries.

CHAPTER III.

PANCREATIC CALCULI.

It has been considered that calculous particles are formed in the pancreas only in exceptional cases. Probably this is true to an extent, as in one series of 1,500 autopsies such concretions were found in but two instances. However, the difficulties of their diagnosis are so great that it has been considered that possibly they exist more frequently than suspected, and that some of the obscure pains of the epigastric region may be due to their presence. In composition, those found have consisted chiefly of carbonate of lime. In size and shape they differ to a considerable extent, but are smaller than calculi of the bile passages.

Symptomatology:—The known cases of pancreatic calculi have been so few in number that their symptoms are not very well known. In those reported, pain of a colicky nature quite similar to gall stone colic has been present. If a stone becomes lodged in one of the ducts, there is obstruction with dilatation resulting, sometimes to such an extent as to be considered a cyst. There have also been reports where injury done by such a calculus was so great that an acute inflammation terminating in suppuration has ensued. And finally the irritation from such a particle may result in the growth of a cancer.

Diagnosis:—Literature reports but five cases that have been diagnosed as pancreatic calculi, and which have been proven by autopsy. It may be suspected where there is severe colicky pain located in the region of the pancreas, where gall stone colic, gastralgia or other painful affections of this region can be eliminated. The only positive diagnostic sign is the finding in the stools of calculi consisting of carbonate of lime.

Treatment:—Usually this could only be palliative, and would consist in the giving of opiates in the manner recommended for gall stone colic. One case has been reported where this condition was suspected, and 1 c. c. of a 1% solution of pilocarpin being given by hypodermic injection three times a day for a week, and the symptoms were relieved. This treatment was given because pilocarpin has been proven to materially increase secretion by the pancreas, and the object was to thus flush out the organ and wash the stones away. Whether the relief resulted from the treatment, of course, cannot be proven.

CHAPTER IV.
CANCER OF THE PANCREAS.

Solid tumors, other than carcinomata, so infrequently affect the pancreas that they may well be left unconsidered. Cancers, however, are probably present in this organ more often than any other form of disease, either benign or malignant; at least such has been the opinion until very recently. Closer study of the organ has caused some to believe that other conditions, especially chronic pancreatitis exists more frequently than has been suspected, and possibly outnumbers the carcinomata. In one series of 11,500 autopsies in the hospital at Milan there were found 132 tumors of the pancreas. Of these 127 were carcinomata, 2 were sarcomata, 1 was syphilitic and 2 were cystic.

Cancer of the pancreas is in the majority of cases secondary to the same condition in some other organ, reaching this gland either by metastasis or by contiguity. However, primary cancer is by no means rare. The growth most frequently starts in the head of the gland, although it may be in the body and in a few cases has originated in the tail. The most frequent form, from a pathological standpoint, is composed largely of fibrous tissue, is nodular, and may be classed as scirrhus. Medullary and gelatinous types are occasionally found. The most common forms are thought to originate from the epithelial cells of the ducts, while those of the uncommon and irregular kinds start from the glandular cells.

The size of the tumor may vary from one presenting only small nodules to one weighing five and one-half pounds, which is the largest one reported. The part of the pancreas not included in the growth may be normal or may be hardened and atrophied as a result of new connective tissue growth. Neighboring organs and tissues are often affected by extension of the growth, and metastases to more distant parts may take place by means of the lymphatics. The ductus communis choledochus, the duct of Wirsung and the pylorus may all be obstructed as a result of compression from the new growth. The result in each of these cases is obvious.

Symptomatology:—The symptoms may be considered from three standpoints:

1.—Those due to disturbances of the pancreas itself.

2.—Those due to pressure of the growth upon neighboring organs.

3.—Those resulting from metastases.

The earlier symptoms seem to be due largely to disturbances of the diseased gland itself. They consist in most cases of a loss of appetite, evidences of indigestion especially in the intestine, emaciation, prostration and pain. The appetite seems especially poor for foods of an albuminous nature, although cases have been seen where the appetite remained good for a considerable period of time. The intestinal indigestion, which is evidently due to interference with the secretion or excretion of the pancreatic juice ,manifests itself by the usual formation of more or less gas, abdominal fulness and distress. In many cases the stools are more bulky than normal, sometimes this being the first indication that the pancreas is affected. These bulky stools follow imperfect digestion of the food, with consequent lessening of its absorption. Upon examination, they may be found to contain an excessive amount of fat, but more commonly their increase of bulk is due to unabsorbed albuminous and vegetable foods. If meat has been eaten there will be found a large number of striated muscle fibres in many cases. Also due to the impaired pancreatic digestion of the carbohydrate elements, sugar may be found in the urine. One observer reports that in a series of 50 cases, sugar was found 13 times. Albumin is also found very frequently, possibly being only func-

tional as a result of imperfect digestion of the albumen
of the food, instead of being due to a nephritis. The emaciation and prostration is caused partly no doubt by the
same cachectic condition which causes these symptoms in
cancer of any part of the body, though also to an extent to
the impairment of the digestion by the disabled functioning of the pancreas. Pain is one of the early symptoms,
usually being constant, though sometimes it appears of a
colicky nature, recurring at frequent intervals. The character of the pain varies in different individuals, some declaring it to be burning, boring, stabbing, drawing or tear-
ing, while in the later stages it may be defined only as
being unbearable. It may be localized in the epigastric
region, or as more frequently happens, it radiates to other
parts, as the chest, lower abdomen, back, loins or in almost any direction. The pain is supposed to be due largely
to pressure or impingement of the nerves constituting the
cœliac plexus, or some of the branches of these nerves.

Symptoms depending upon pressure of the growth on
neighboring organs depend of course upon the direction
taken by the tumor. It may compress the pylorus, causing
the symptoms described in the chapter upon that subject.
The bile duct is pressed upon in quite a number of cases,
resulting in a jaundice especially characterized by its tendency to continue for a long time. The liver may suffer
from presence of the growth, its functions being interfered
with to some extent. Ascites may develop as a result of
pressure upon the portal vein. If any of the above mentioned organs which are in relationship with the pancreas
become affected with the growth as they usually do in the
course of time, symptoms more appropriately studied in
the diseases of these organs arise, to be added to those already present from the diseased pancreas.

Symptoms caused by development of cancers in distant organs as a result of metastases, are also to be studied under different subjects than the one now under consideration. The organs most apt to be affected in this manner are the liver, skin, heart, lungs, pleura, large intestine and, indeed in almost any part of the body. Sometimes a condition of general carcinosis develops. It may be difficult to determine which is the primary location of the growth in some cases.

Diagnosis:—The points from which a diagnosis may often be made are, the pain as described in the symptomatology, the emaciation and cachexia, the stationary jaundice, the bulky stools with possibly the microscopical and chemical findings as mentioned which show interference with the pancreatic digestion, possibly the sugar in the urine and the presence of the tumor. This last sign, the presence of a tumor, is demonstrable in only a limited number of cases, probably not more than 25%. Even when found, it is not of very much value from a diagnostic standpoint, except when considered in conjunction with the other signs, especially the laboratory findings. In the first place it is extremely difficult to determine that the tumor is certainly of the pancreas instead of the stomach, duodenum, gall bladder, liver, colon, peritoneum or other part. In the second place even if positive that it is of the pancreas, it cannot generally be said to be cancer instead of inflammatory or cystic. In reality a majority of cases will have to pass without our being positive that this disease exists. The fatty and albuminous stools are by no means universally present. Diabetes and tumor are to be found in only about one-fourth of the cases, and when present are not conclusive evidence, and all the other symptoms may be due to other conditions. The deep,

chronic and progressive jaundice is possibly as characteristic as any symptom, especially if a distended gall bladder can be outlined, though this condition may be absent.

Prognosis:—Owing to the difficulty in determining when
the disease commenced, it is generally impossible to say
how long the patient may live after inception of the
growth. Cases have died within six weeks after decided
symptoms have begun, at other times six months to a year
has elapsed.

Treatment:—This can be of but slight avail. Efforts
should be made to nourish the patient as well as possible,
by mouth as long as the pylorus and duodenum are patulous, by rectum after this stage. The use of a pancreatic
extract has been recommended in disease of the pancreas.
Possibly some slight benefit may be obtained in this manner, but in reality artificial ferments are chiefly of theoretical rather than of practical value in diseases of this
organ as well as in diseases of the stomach. Pain must
generally be alleviated at least during the later stages. For
this purpose some preparation of opium will in most cases
have to be employed. Operative measures have been resorted to in a few isolated instances, but assistance from
this source does not seem to offer very much hope of success.

Part VII.– Diseases of the Peritoneum.

CHAPTER I.

ACUTE PERITONITIS.

Inflammation of the peritoneum is probably always caused by bacteria. In the past it has been supposed that traumatism, certain chemical irritants or foreign bodies might cause the condition. But in reality such causes quite likely act only as a means by which bacteria may gain entrance, or form a fertile field for their greater activity. Bacteria may reach the peritoneal cavity by any of the following routes:

1.—By extension through the parietes.

2.—By means of the blood.

3.—From an infection arising within the peritoneal cavity.

Examples of the first method are, a penetrating wound through the abdominal walls, extension of an empyæma or lung abscess through the diaphragm, extension of a puerperal infection through the walls of the uterus or tubes, and possibly a few other conditions. Bacteria circulating in the blood current probably never cause peritonitis unless there is previously some injury or irritation of the membrane. In fact, cases arising from either of these two methods are comparatively rare. In at least 95% of all attacks the infection occurs by means of disease of some of the organs of which the peritoneum composes the external coat. Such organs are the appendix, the pylorus, the gall bladder and bile ducts and the female genital organs.

313

There are several varieties of bacteria which may produce the condition under consideration. The bacillus coli communis is the one most frequently active, although the frequent presence of this type in superior numbers may be partly due to the fact that it is able to multiply with greater rapidity than many other kinds, and possibly in instances where some other bacillus was primarily at fault, their numbers have been reduced by the surpassing activities of the colon bacilli. In fact one investigator believes that the staphylococcus albus in most cases is the one which instigates the trouble and the colon bacilli only act secondarily. At least the staphylococci, the streptococci and the bacillus pyocyaneus are frequently present. Sometimes the typhoid bacillus, the pneumococcus and the gonococcus are to be found.

Pathology:—Considered from the standpoint of the amount of peritoneal surface involved, this disease may be classified as:

1.—Diffuse.

2.—Circumscribed.

Into which of these classes a given case develops, depends upon the virulence of the bacilli, the rapidity with which the bacteria gain access to the cavity of the peritoneum and the resisting power of the individual. If the bacteria are not particularly destructive, if the parts are kept at rest so that the rapidity of their access is lessened, if the process giving rise to them is chronic in nature, or if the resisting power to this particular type of bacilli is high, then there is apt to develop a fibrinous or adhesive peritonitis in advance of the more severe inflammation. This will result in adhesions by which the bacteria are held in check, and the process becomes circumscribed. On the other hand, if these conditions do not exist, the infectious material spreads in all directions and the entire inner surface of the peritoneum may become inflamed.

The degree or severity of the inflammation varies in the different stages, and depends to a great extent upon the same factors which are of importance in determining as to whether it is diffuse or circumscribed. At first there is congestion only, advancing soon to the production of a fibrinous exudate. If conditions are favorable, it may not progress beyond this stage, or it may advance to the formation of a serous or fibrinous exudation. In cases operated upon early this is often found to be present. If not operated upon or otherwise checked, this stage changes to one where there is suppuration in the majority of cases, although exceptionally there will be gangrene.

Symptomatology:—In the vast majority of cases in which the infection gains access by way of some diseased intra-abdominal organ, the symptoms will depend to a great extent upon the organ primarily affected. For instance, the symptoms mentioned when considering appendicitis, cholecystitis, gastric ulcer, etc., will first be present, and upon perforation, the peritoneal cavity will become involved and the symptoms pertaining to this membrane itself will begin.

Usually the first symptom to make its appearance when the peritoneum becomes involved is pain. It is generally felt throughout the abdomen, but sometime during the course of the disease, will be felt more particularly in the region from which the infection originates, except in occasional cases of fulminating peritonitis where the entire abdomen becomes inflamed before the period of general pain subsides. Such a condition is more apt to follow perforation of the stomach, duodenum or gall bladder, and materially adds to the difficulty of the diagnosis. Very shortly after the beginning of the pain there is nearly always nausea and vomiting. The vomiting is persistent and causes great aggravation of the pain. These two symptoms are so pronounced and give rise to so great distress that an appearance of collapse with the cold sweat, pinched countenance, and general expression commonly spoken of as the Hippocratic countenance is present. The patient seeks to find a position which will relieve the suffering and sinks down deeply in the bed flexing the thighs on the abdomen. The abdominal muscles, acting automatically, become rigid in an attempt to protect the deeper lying organs; the abdomen is therefore retracted until the later stage when gaseous distention has become so great that there is marked abdominal bulging. Upon pressure, there is extreme tenderness, usually most intense over the seat of the original lesion. In typhoid fever with perforation and general peritonitis, the sensorium has generally been so benumbed by the original disease that the symptoms resulting from the peritonitis are less prominent, and unless one is careful may escape notice.

As mentioned before, if the bacteria possess but a mild degree of virulence, if their escape into the peritoneal cavity is slow, or if the patient's resisting power is good, adhesions may form around the zone of infection, limiting it in extent and giving rise to the so-called circumscribed peritonitis. In such a case the symptoms are generally milder. However, as to whether such adhesions are forming or not is often a matter difficult to decide, possibly because people differ so much as regards the ease with which symptoms are produced. The severity and rapidity of onset of some of the symptoms will also depend to an extent upon the portion of the abdominal cavity in which the infection has its origin. The peritoneum of the upper part of the abdomen seems to absorb the toxic products of a suppurative peritonitis much more rapidly than does the pelvic portion. The reason for this is not positively known, but it has been suggested that the up and down movements of the diaphragm may act somewhat as a pump, and by its alternating suction and pressure the rapidity of absorption is increased. Ordinarily there is a rapid increase of the leucocytes in the blood, as a result of the effort made by the natural forces to antagonize the infectious products. This so-called leucocytosis was formerly thought to be an index by which the severity of the infection could be determined, and to offer a means by which it was possible to differentiate between the circumscribed and the diffuse varieties. It is now considered, however, that the proportion of polynuclear cells to the entire number of white ones is the important point, and that if such polynuclears are in proportionately high percentage the attack was a severe one. Of still greater import is it, if the entire number of leucocytes is but slightly increased, and the polynuclears are present in a considerable higher percentage than normal. The interpretation drawn is that the attack is not only a severe one, but that the patient's abilities for resistance are at a low point.

The pulse rate is generally rapid, the volume is small and the artery is apt to have a wiry feeling. The temperature varies; at first as a result of shock it may be subnormal, later there may be fever. Chill, high temperature and sweat are apt to irregularly alternate

Diagnosis:—The three symptoms of importance in determining acute peritonitis are pain, nausea and muscular rigidity. When these symptoms are present with a preceding history indicating any of the lesions which have been mentioned as instigators of the condition such a diag-

nosis is generally warranted. The diseases from which it
will have to be differentiated are intestinal obstruction,
ruptured ectopic pregnancy, Dietl's crisis, acute pancreatitis, diaphragmatic pleurisy, mesenteric thrombosis and
the abdominal crises of locomotor ataxia. This is too long
a list to consider differentially, but these diseases should
be kept in mind when acute abdominal symptoms are present.

In addition to determining the presence of peritonitis,
an attempt should be made to decide as to whether it is
diffuse or circumscribed. The features of importance are
the severity and extent of the pain, the amount of vomiting, the degree of muscular rigidity, the extent of collapse, the temperature, the appearance of the countenance,
the character of the pulse, the extent and degree of tenderness and the results of the blood count. Many times,
however, in spite of attention to all these points it will tax
one's shrewdness to the uttermost to arrive at a correct
conclusion.

Prognosis:—Acute diffuse peritonitis has always been
considered an extremely dangerous condition, but owing
to certain changes in the technique of its treatment within
very recent years a much more hopeful prognosis may be
offered, provided appropriate treatment is instituted at a
sufficiently early period. Acute circumscribed peritonitis
is a much less severe affair, although careful diagnosis and
treatment are also of great importance in this form.

Treatment:—Treatment of the two forms, diffuse and
circumscribed, differs so materially in some respects that
they will be considered separately. The treatment for the
former variety should be positively surgical, and should
be instituted at the earliest possible moment. Arising as
it generally does from perforation of some of the organs

covered by peritoneum, there is no means of escape for the bacteria, and it is only in rare instances that the resisting powers are able to cope with the infection unless drainage is instituted. However, there are certain adjuvants of a medical nature which are so important that the fate of the patient generally depends upon their proper application in addition to the surgical procedures. Of first importance, is as nearly absolute rest as possible. If necessary to get the patient to a hospital, it should be done as easily as possible. The position of the patient both in bed or while in an invalid carriage is important, for the reason mentioned in the symptomatology, that absorption is more rapid in the upper abdomen than in the lower. Therefore a nearly erect sitting posture, the so-called Fowler position should be employed. By this means pus or other fluids have a tendency to gravitate toward the pelvis where absorption is less rapid. No attempt should be made to stimulate bowel movement, but instead peristalsis should if possible be exhibited. This may be done by allowing absolutely nothing to be taken into the stomach, by cold applications and by rest in bed. If there is persistent vomiting, systematic lavage should be performed. The great improvement recently instituted in the treatment of this condition is the Murphy enteroclysis. This is particularly applicable after the abdomen has been opened, but is also useful before this has been done. It consists in suspending some container, as a fountain syringe, just high enough above the patient, usually six to twelve inches, so that a normal salt solution will flow into the bowel through a rubber tube and a specially constructed rectal tip at a rate of one to two pints an hour. This is kept up almost constantly, keeping the solution at about body temperature by means of hot water bags placed around the rubber tube, or otherwise. Various improved devices have been invented for performing this treatment, but their absence should be no excuse for not employing it, as it can be done very well by means of the ordinary fountain syringe. Fluid going into the bowel thus slowly is all absorbed, thus relieving the patient's distress to a great extent, but particularly increasing his resisting power, promoting elimination of toxins by the natural emunctories, and after drainage is instituted very materially increasing the flushing given to the peritoneum.

Authorities do not agree as to the advisability of using morphia in diffuse peritonitis. It has the advantage of limiting peristalsis and by relieving the pain probably reduces the amount of shock. On the other hand it masks symptoms, promotes intestinal retention, thus increasing toxic absorption, and it is said that it diminishes the number of leucocytes, thus acting against the protective forces of the body. It seems that each case should be considered separately as regards the use of this drug, depending upon whether the diagnosis has been made, whether a decision for operation has been made, and the necessity for delay until suitable arrangements have been made.

The treatment of circumscribed peritonitis depends upon its extent and upon the nature of exudate that has formed. If there is only a plastic product resulting in adhesions, delay may be allowed, or possibly no radical treatment may be needed. If pus has formed, it should be evacuated the same as an abscess in any other part of the body. The question as to when is the best time to operate, is however, one that may need some study. If the process does not seem to be spreading, delay is advisable until the limiting adhesions have become firm. If spreading, or there are signs that pus is leaking from the circumscribed area, it is better to operate at once. Rest in bed, relief of pain and vomiting, limiting of peristalsis and abstinence from food and drink should be insisted upon in each case, but position and enteroclysis may not be advisable in all cases.

Remedies for acute peritonitis may be useful when the process is limited to an area about an inflamed appendix or a pyloric ulcer, or other lesion of that kind, however, when perforation has occurred and the infection is free in the cavity of this membrane, remedies cannot be of any very decided benefit, and no time should be spent in waiting for their action.

CHAPTER II.

CHRONIC PERITONITIS.

Chronic inflammation of the peritoneum may be considered under three classes:

1.—Adhesive peritonitis.

2.—Exudative peritonitis.

3.—Proliferative peritonitis.

Chronic adhesive peritonitis may be present as a termination of some acute inflammation or may be chronic from the beginning. The former type is much more common than the latter, and is initiated by some such process as appendicitis, gastric ulcer, bile tract inflammations and diseases of the female genitalia. The earlier symptoms have been described under the subject of acute peritonitis. During this stage there is a formation of plastic materials which result in binding different organs or coils of intestines together, or the organs and intestines may become adhered to the peritoneal coat lining the abdominal cavity. The acute symptoms finally subside and the condition remains as a chronic peritonitis.

The second form of adhesive peritonitis begins without acute symptoms though the pathology and symptoms are similar to the other variety. This is more apt to begin in the region of the liver or spleen, although it is sometimes found lower in the abdomen, involving the intestines.

The symptoms of adhesive peritonitis may be caused in either one of two ways. Bands connecting two surfaces may be so placed that a loop of intestine becomes constricted in such a manner that obstruction is produced. This condition of affairs has been sufficiently considered under the subject of intestinal obstruction. The other and more common symptoms are chronic in nature and a determination of their origin is many times difficult. They may be manifested as a persistent colicky pain, rendering life miserable. There may be flatulence, constipation, distention and other symptoms of indigestion, or the symptoms may be of a nervous nature, especially neurasthenic. There are undoubtedly many cases going the round of phy sicians, quacks, patent medicines and faith healers, trying to obtain relief from nervous and digestive disorders, in whom chronic peritoneal adhesions cause all the trouble.

The condition is notably difficult to diagnose, because the symptoms are exactly the same as may be present from other conditions, either organic or functional in nature. There is nothing which can be detected by means of physical diagnosis. But, if in a case presenting the symptoms mentioned, a careful examination fails to reveal any organic disease, if treatment for neurasthenia or other functional diseases thoroughly applied fails to give relief, and especially if careful study of the history of the case reveals attacks in the past which may be interpreted as being any of the acute affections mentioned as instigators of adhesive peritonitis, one is justified in suspecting this condition. If the symptoms are severe enough to warrant it, the treatment indicated for peritoneal adhesions should be employed. This treatment is surgical in nature, and consists in entering the abdomen and loosening the adhesions. Many times individuals who have been practically wrecks, will show signs of improvement almost as soon as they recover from the anæsthetic, and will quickly return to a state of excellent health.

Chronic exudative peritonitis is found especially as a result of cancer or tuberculosis. Cancer of the peritoneum is in the majority of cases secondary, and may occur as a metastasis from cancer of almost any part of the body, but especially when the disease affects some other organ of the abdomen or pelvis. Cases which were undoubtedly primary in origin have however been reported. Whether primary or secondary, there are generally a number of nodular growths of various sizes. There is puckering of the membrane, and a considerable amount of associated inflammation which gives rise to the effusion or exudation. This is often somewhat tinged with blood. Adhesions may also be present, if so they are generally in the form of bands instead of a diffuse character.

The symptoms of cancer of the peritoneum outside of the ascites are not very prominent. There may be some pain, possibly fever, and if the effusion is not too great the nodules may be felt. The inguinal glands are often enlarged. The diagnosis may generally be made by these symptoms developing in one who is subject to a cancerous growth in some other part of the body. When primary, the diagnosis is more difficult but may possibly be made by the symptoms mentioned, together with the presence of the cancerous cachexia, emaciation and enlargement of neighboring glands.

Tuberculosis of the peritoneum may be associated with the disease in some other part of the body, or may be present independently. It is manifested in some one of three forms:

1.—The miliary type in which the effusion is sero-fibrinous or bloody.

2.—Where there is a development of true tubercles which have a tendency to caseate or ulcerate, and in which the exudate is purulent or sero-purulent.

3.—A fibroid tuberculosis in which the tubercles are hard and fibrous. In this form the exudate is serous and scanty or possibly absent, and there may be some adhesions present.

This affection is apt to start in the neighborhood of the Fallopian tubes or the prostate or in hernial sacs. Other abdominal diseases seem to predispose to this condition, especially cirrhosis of the liver.

The mode of onset varies to a great extent. Sometimes there will be no symptoms, and the condition will be found accidentally, at other times there will be such a violent onset that enteritis or other acute disease may be diagnosed. There may be fever, abdominal tenderness and tympanitis. The exudate is seldom large, is sometimes bloody, and may be sacculated. The omentum may become so puckered as to simulate a tumor, and at other times the intestinal coils may appear so massed and hardened as to appear as a new growth. The intestinal walls are generally thickened, and the mesenteric glands enlarged.

The diagnosis may be quite difficult. When masses due to the thickened omentum or intestines are found they may be mistaken for other forms of tumor, and where the exudate exists in the form of a saccular cyst, it is very often mistaken for an ovarian cyst. If tubercular lesions can be found in the lungs or in other parts of the body they may assist very materially in making the diagnosis. If there are no other tubercular foci, the general physical condition may not be of much assistance in making a diagnosis, because quite frequently at such times the general health is excellent. In case of doubt use may be made of some of the tuberculin tests; using it either by injection subcutaneously, by inunction of the skin or by instillation into the conjunctivæ.

Chronic proliferative peritonitis is characterized by a considerable thickening of the membrane. There may be slight adhesions, but they are not apt to be marked. It is often associated with sclerotic conditions of some of the other abdominal organs, as the liver, the stomach, the cæcum, the spleen or the first part of the colon. The thickening may be universal or in patches. The omentum, the mesentery or some other portion may become almost cartilaginous in density owing to the extreme development of the fibrous elements. At such times they are greatly shortened, and in case of the mesentery the suspended intestines are so drawn up toward the back that they appear as a hard ball. This affection is comparatively rare, there being no particular cause known that has an influence in its production, although alcoholism and syphilis have been accused of such an influence. Its treatment is extremely unsatisfactory.

CHAPTER III.
ASCITES.

Definition:—An accumulation of a watery fluid in the cavity of the peritoneum.

Etiology:—It may be due to local causes such as—

1.—Obstruction to the portal circulation either by compression of the terminal branches in the liver as in cirrhosis, or by pressure on the vein itself as by a tumor of some other organ.

2.—Chronic inflammation of the peritoneum, especially cancerous or tubercular.

3.—A thrombus may form in the portal vein, resulting in a serous exudate in the peritoneal cavity.

4.—Tumors of the abdomen which exert pressure on some portion of the peritoneal membrane.

It may also be a part of a general dropsical condition caused by such diseases as cardiac obstruction or insufficiency, Bright's disease, emphysema, pulmonary sclerosis or in general hydræmic conditions of the blood.

Diagnosis:—As it is but a symptom of some of the affections mentioned in the etiology, its diagnosis has to do not only with determining that it is ascites, but also in determining which of these lesions is its causative factor.

Inspection shows a protuberant abdomen, the location of the greatest amount of bulging depending upon the position of the patient. For instance if lying upon the side, gravity will carry the fluid to that side and the other one will appear somewhat flattened. If there is a large exudate, the skin will appear tense, possibly with some bulging of the umbilicus. In some cases the superficial veins will be distended, possibly varicosed. When this condition exists about the navel, it has been called the caput Medusæ.

Palpation employed properly will in most cases detect a fluctuation. The best method is to have a second party hold the ulnar margin of his hand firmly on the linea alba, while the examiner holds the palm of one hand against one side of the abdomen and with the other hand strikes sharply against the other side. The fluctuation wave will then be felt quite distinctly by the first hand.

Percussion, with the patient flat on the back reveals a dullness on both flanks, while there is tympanitis in the median line as a result of the intestines floating to the top of the fluid. If the patient now rolls to one side there will be dullness at the lower side, while the tympanitis will change to the upper side. This sign may not be applicable unless there is, at least a quart of fluid present.

Conditions with which ascites may be confounded are a distended bladder and an ovarian cyst. The former may be differentiated, of course, by the passing of a catheter. In an ovarian cyst, the chief dullness is at the top, with the patient in the reclining position, and the tympanitis is at the flanks where the intestines have been pushed by the tumor. In ascites the fluid seldom has a specific gravity above 1,015, while in ovarian cyst it is generally above that point. In ascites due to anæmia, Bright's disease or cardias affections, the fluid is usually light, or straw colored, while in cirrhosis of the liver it is darker. In tubercular and cancerous peritonitis it is bloody. Occasionally it appears chylous or milky, such instances usually being associated with cancer of the peritoneum, although when existing only to a mild degree it may be found in other conditions.

Treatment:—This depends to a considerable extent upon the causative lesion, and is described in the chapters given to those subjects. However, if treatment for the process which gives rise to the ascites is not sufficient to take care of this symptom, some method especially for its relief may be employed. Strong cathartics, such as sulphate of magnesia, a large dose with but a little water taken before breakfast, will sometimes suffice.   Bitartrate of potash, preferably taken with jalap will often reduce or entirely remove fluid from the peritoneal cavity.   Apocynum or infusion of digitalis may be useful in nephritic or cardiac dropsy of the abdomen.   If however an immediate relief is desired, better success may be obtained by tapping. This is a simple and comparatively safe process, and if the ascites has reached very large proportions is the most satisfactory method of relief.

Part VIII.—Abdominal Splanchnoptosis.

CHAPTER I.

Definition :—A prolapse of the abdominal organs as a result of relaxation of their ligaments and of the abdominal walls.

Etiology :—As a predisposing cause may be mentioned a poorly developed osseous system. In some skeletons, the depressions in which organs rest, and the prominences to which ligaments are attached are imperfectly formed. Or the bones comprising the trunk of the body may be so arranged that a shallow abdomen is produced, with possibly an unduly downward slanting of the anterior surface of the posterior abdominal wall. Such imperfect development and construction may be congenital or it may be due to rachitis in early life. Because of the abnormal conditions mentioned, the organs in the abdomen are more than normally dependent upon their ligamentous attachments. This increased dependence and accompanying strain is inclined to cause a prolapse, and then if some exciting cause arises to weaken the vitality and strength of the body tissues, or to decrease the adipose tissue which may have been so located as to form some support to the organs, the tendency to prolapse is increased. A lessening of the adipose tissue seems to have considerable influence, especially if there is a marked decrease within a short period of time. It evidently acts not only in removing a part of the support to the organs, but also in causing a loss in the amount of intra-abdominal tension.

As examples of the exciting causes which produce a loss of vitality and of fat, may be mentioned the acute fevers. Chronic diseases of a wasting or prostrating nature act in the same. manner.   A history of chlorosis occurring about the period of puberty may often be obtained from women, who in later life suffer from splanchnoptosis.   Rickets in childhood as a predisposing cause and chlorosis at puberty as an exciting cause are frequently associated in these cases.   Affections characterized by severe coughing have been declared to act as causes.   For instance, whooping cough or an attack of bronchitis which continues for some time and is accompanied with severe attacks of coughing. Strains from other sources, as lifting heavy weights, may act in the same way. Falls upon the buttocks may have the same effect, due to the sudden jar. Women who have frequent pregnancies are especially prone to splanchnoptosis.   This undoubtedly arises from the stretching and weakening of the abdominal muscles as well as from the prostration and emaciation which is apt to be produced by the repeated pregnancies and the ensuing lactation. Tight lacing is undobutedly a potent cause in many cases. Some writers have considered this the chief and almost neces- ary cause. This however, cannot be true, for if the con- dition is looked for carefully enough it will often be found in women who have never worn a corset.   Abdominal splanchnoptosis is found much more frequently in women than in men, due probably to greater frailty of the osseous system and muscular development, to their habit of wear- ing corsets and suspending the weight of their skirts from the waist, and to their child bearing.

Symptomatology:—In a patient suffering from the con- dition under consideration it is often difficult to determine which symptoms are due to the displaced abdominal organs. Looking at the matter in a conservative manner, it would seem that some of the symptoms which are often present should possibly be considered as a part of the same general atonic condition which permits the prolapse, instead of being considered as due to the prolapse. The anæmic and neurasthenic symptoms which often exist are examples of this class. Yet looked at in another way, it would seem that these same symptoms are to an extent at least caused by the splanchnoptosis, because they may be so much more thoroughly remedied after means have been employed to correct the visceral displacements.

In whatever relationship they may be considered the symptoms which are most frequently observed are quite characteristic. The patient is apt to be slender, rather narrow chested, and a peculiarity of structure which is present in nearly all cases is that the tenth rib, like the eleventh and twelfth, is not attached to the sternum. In the epigastric region there is very often a depression, while the lower part of the abdomen protrudes and sags more than normal. The patient tires easily, and any work which necessitates a stooping posture or a twisting movement of the body is especially exhausting. There is often a backache, or at least a dragging sensation which is especially prominent in the dorsal region. This is felt when on the feet and is much relieved by assuming the recumbent position. There is apt to be an undue irritability of temper or else depression and melancholia. Digestive symptoms are numerous, especially flatulence and constipation.

Considering the symptoms more particularly in connection with the individual organs it may be said that those arising from a fallen stomach are due largely to the resulting stagnation of food within its cavity, and are very similar to those mentioned in the chapter on motor insufficiency. In fact a prolapsed stomach is very often a part of motor insufficiency. Belching of gas, pyrosis and a distended sensation especially after eating are generally present. The secretions of the stomach may be normal, excessive or deficient. Probably in a majority of cases they are excessive, and then the symptoms of hyperchlorhydria are added. On inspection the outlines of the greater curvature of the stomach may often be seen below its normal location. It is of considerable importance to try and locate the lesser curvature, for if it is found to be lower than it should be the case is one of gastroptosis; if not, and still the greater curvature is descended, it is dilatation. By tapping with the tips of the fingers over the region of the stomach after food or drink has been taken, a splashing sound may be elicited in most cases. Some writers attach much importance to this splashing or so-called succussion sound, and believe that when present it is sufficient upon which to base a diagnosis of atony of the gastric walls. In testing for this sound, it is important to determine beyond doubt that it originates in the stomach, inasmuch as the same sound may often be obtained from the intestines, especially from the transverse colon. When it can be produced on a level with the umbilicus, or even lower than that point, it is difficult to determine whether it is from prolapsed stomach or from the colon. A good way to decide is to fill the stomach with air forced through a stomach tube by means of an atomizer bulb. Percussion, or even inspection will then show the location of the greater curvature. These patients often have a pronounced pulsation in the epigastric region or slightly below, in the upper part of the hypogastric portion. This pulsation may also be felt by the examining hand, and is produced by the abdominal aorta which has been dragged forward by the pendent viscera. It has sometimes been mistaken for aneurysm of the aorta. It may be differentiated however by its lacking the expansile character of pulsation.

The transverse colon is often prolapsed, especially in its middle portion. This may be so marked that it assumes the position of the letter V. It is caused partly by a relaxed mesocolon and partly from the pressure by a prolapsed stomach upon its superior margin. Its existence interferes with a free passage of fæces, and marked constipation is apt to result. In some cases, palpation over the abdomen in the course of the transverse colon gives the sensation of a band or cord. This condition has been called corde colique. By some it is thought to be due to the colon being put on a stretch, by others it is thought to be the pancreas dragged forward by the more superficial organs.

Of all abdominal organs susceptible to the condition of splanchnoptosis, the kidney, because of its peculiar shape and firm texture, is the one most easily palpated. Because of this reason more has been said about it than of the other organs. With many, a movable or floating kidney is all that is considered in this line. Its importance is undoubted, but its existence is probably no more common than is the same condition of the other organs. Therefore suturing the kidney in place as has been so often recommended, and leaving the other viscera untouched, seems woefully illogical. The right kidney is the one most often loose, although it may sometimes be the left one; in exceptional cases both of them are more movable than normal. The degree of movability varies from one which may just be detected, to that where the organ may be carried to the opposite side of the median line and down into the inguinal region. The best way to diagnose a movable kidney is to have the patient lie comfortably on the back with the legs flexed. For the right kidney the examiner places his left hand firmly against the patient's back in the region of the kidney, and the right hand lightly over the abdomen in front of the organ. The patient is then instructed. to take a deep abdominal inspiration. As expiration begins, the right hand is firmly pressed downward toward the left hand. If the kidney is movable it may be felt as it slips backward into place, or, as said above, if it is very movable it may be so grasped that it can be held out of its place and even moved about the abdomen. Experience in making this examination will result in proficiency, until one, especially if his work is largely with digestive diseases, will begin to think that nearly all women have a loose right kidney.

The kidney is not apt to have symptoms pertaining to itself, although in rare instances the ureter may become so twisted or kinked that interference is produced with the passage of the urine through this canal. At such times severe colicky pains are produced. The name of Dietl's crisis is given to this phenomenon. Occasionally the urine may be held back to such an extent as to cause a dilatation of the pelvis of the kidney, a condition called hydronephrosis. Other symptoms which are caused by a movable right kidney pertain especially to the digestive and nervous systems. The location and attachments of this kidney are such that when displaced downward it carries with it to some extent the duodenum and the hepatic flexure of the colon. By thus dragging on the duodenum its lumen and its connection with the stomach are somewhat obstructed. As a result the food is delayed in its exit from the stomach and this gives rise to the symptoms mentioned when considering gastroptosis. In other words, the nephroptosis probably has some influence in increasing an already existing prolapsed stomach. In dragging down the colon, the direction and channel of that organ is modified in such a manner as to interfere with the passage of the fœces. Besides these effects, the up and down movement of the kidney, as when walking, or especially when stooping, causes a friction against portions of the intestine, and in this way also interferes with the proper performance of its functions. In what manner a loose kidney acts upon the nervous system to cause symptoms, is not as easily understood. Probably the unnatural movements and the dragging upon the attachments have some effect. The general stigmata of which the nephroptosis is one indication, is quite likely manifested in the nervous system in such a manner as to make it unduly impressionable to irritating influences. The nervous symptoms are generally of the neurasthenic and hysterical type. There are patients, however, who have good general health, with no indication of any abnormal condition, yet in whom if a careful examination is made, a movable kidney may be found. Evidently such people have sufficient nerve stamina to resist the effects of the peculiarity. In such cases, it is the part of policy to refrain from telling them of this condition, as the information will sometimes act upon their minds in such a way as to help in instituting symptoms. Even in those who already have symptoms, it is better to say nothing about the movable kidney, provided the necessary treatment can be carried out without giving this as a reason. The mental effect of knowing about such an abnormality is often deleterious.

Other abdominal organs which may be prolapsed are the liver and spleen. It seems however that such a condition is much more rare than of the stomach, colon and kidney. For this reason, and also because there are no marked symptoms which differ from those already mentioned, no further consideration will be made in connection with these organs.

Diagnosis:—One may suspect an abdominal splanchnoptosis in an individual presenting the skeletal appearance described in the etiology. This suspicion may be increased by the presence of the various digestive and nervous symptoms mentioned. It may be confirmed by the physical signs of the various organs, which have been given. For the stomach there is the succussion sound, the prolapsed organ upon disténding with air or gas, or its lowered position seen upon using the gastrodiaphane. The transverse colon may also be outlined when distended with air or fluid. The kidney may be palpated in its abnormal positions by employing the bi-manual method of examination as described.

Prognosis:—This is not a condition which is dangerous to life, but when once established it is extremely difficult to eradicate. However the associated or resulting symptoms may be very much improved, or possibly entirely relieved by proper treatment.

Treatment:—When applicable, the best treatment which can be employed in this class of cases, is for the patient to become pregnant. In order to make pregnancy of use it must be carefully managed. Women having this affection generally have more than the usual amount of distress during the first few weeks after conception; that is, there are many nervous symptoms with much nausea and vomiting. Later when the uterus has sufficiently increased in size to reach up into the abdomen these symptoms will disappear. The support furnished by the growing uterus relieves the peritoneal ligaments of part of the weight which it is their function to sustain. As a result, · the nervous strain is lessened, the appetite improves, nausea, flatulence and other signs of indigestion disappear, and these women will often say that they feel better during the latter half of pregnancy that at any other time of their lives. Now unless particular care is exercised, the relief experienced at this time will continue for only a variable length of time after parturition, then there is a recurrence. The care of the baby, lactation and the loss of the temporary support furnished by the enlarged uterus results in a return to the former condition. This in many cases may be prevented if attention is given to certain details. During the last four or five months of pregnancy, when they are feeling at their best an especial effort should be made by means of forced feeding, recreation and general hygienic care to build up as much flesh and strength as possible. When labor ensues, it should be made as short and easy as is consistent, limiting shock, exhaustion and hæmorrhage to the lowest possible point. No attempt should be made to nurse the baby, as cow's milk can be modified to take care of its nutrition, and the mother should not be exhausted by the drain of lactation. A rather longer period than usual should be spent in bed, during which time and afterwards an especial effort should be made to keep up a high state of nutrition by plenty of food, fresh air, proper elimination, and other hygienic means. When the mother does get up from the lying-in period, abdominal support should be furnished by an elastic bandage or adhesive bands applied according to the method described later in this article. She should also be cautioned against heavy lifting, reaching or other work which might cause any undue strain upon the abdominal organs.

The above method of treatment has given excellent and lasting results in cases where it was applicable. But evidently when splanchnoptosis is present in men, unmarried women and in some women who are married this line of treatment is not practicable. It has been said by some writers that many girls who are sufferers from chlorosis until marriage, and then who improve so rapidly after marriage and pregnancy have occurred, are cured in this manner. In reality they were victims of splanchnoptosis until cured by this method, but if circumstances are not favorable, they will not be permanently cured, and sometimes are made worse after the temporary improvement, as a result of the factors mentioned in the etiology.

When for obvious reasons a case cannot be treated by pregnancy, other means may be employed which give quite good results. If, as so frequently happens, the patient is emaciated, anæmic and neurasthenic, the well known Weir Mitchell rest treatment is excellent. It must be carried out thoroughly as outlined in the chapter on treatment of the nervous gastric disorders. An especial effort should be made to have the patient gain weight, as in this manner the fat formed in the omentum, around the ligamentous attachments of the various organs and on the abdominal walls will materially assist in maintaining intra-abdominal tension and thus help in supporting the viscera. After a sufficient period of rest in bed, care should be exercised in getting up, selected exercises may be employed in an effort to build up the tonicity of the abdominal and general muscular systems, and all means at one's disposal should be employed to improve the health and to keep the mind as cheerful as possible. An especial effort should be made to impress upon the patient the fact that the object for which the treatment was instituted has been accomplished. As said in the etiology, if these people think there is a displaced kidney or other organ it often affects them deleteriously. So at this time their minds should be relieved from any such anxiety. If for any reason the abdominal muscles seem so flaccid that it is impossible to develop them by exercises or other means, it may be well to have the patients wear bandages, but they should do it with the idea that it is not necessary for purposes of treating any condition present, but merely to prevent a recurrence.

There will be other cases, in fact in practice these will probably constitute the largest class of all, in whom neither of the methods of treatment outlined so far, can be employed. For these sufferers it is necessary to employ whatever seems best adapted in the individual case. Usually some form of abdominal support will be of chief consequence. Many forms of bandages and other appliances have been devised, some giving particular attention to one feature, some to another. In fact none of them are the best one for all cases. If a woman has a fairly prominent abdomen, that is when in the erect position if there is a considerable protuberance between the anterior borders of their iliac bones, simply the plain elastic bandage, lacing up in the back will generally be all that is necessary, if properly applied. In those who are emaciated to such an extent that their abdomen is nearly flat at this point, such a bandage will be of but limited value. In such an individual, adhesive plaster may be employed in such a manner as to give much more support, and in all cases it may be used with certainly as much and possibly more benefit. The great objection to it however, is that it irritates the skin somewhat, although this may be partly overcome by using a good grade of the zinc oxide plaster. It also interferes with free bathing, and in women of æsthetic habits seems unclean and obnoxious. These features may be overcome to some extent by putting on a new plaster at frequent intervals, thus allowing opportunities for bathing and keeping the skin free from irritation. To apply this dressing the patient should be lying flat on the back, possibly if an aggravated case, on an inclined plane with the head at the lower end. The abdomen and hips should be exposed, with no clothing whatever in the way to adhere to the plaster and interfere with its application. Then with a roll of zinc oxide plaster, about two and one-half inches in width begin above the pubes and as near to them as possible without its being on the hair at this point, and apply in such a manner that the plaster will pass upward and to the right, over the crest of the ilium and around to the back, slightly crossing to the left of the spine, on a level with the center of the dorsal region. Beginning again at the same place over the pubes, another strip is placed on the left side in exactly the same way. If experience shows that the individual can comfortably bear them so, these strips should be placed quite firmly, using some upward tension as they are put in place. Then beginning on the left side over the region of the gluteus muscle, and on a level with the superior margin of the pubic hair, another strip is placed transversely to the same point on the right side, also drawing it quite firmly. Usually it is better to apply a second strip immediately above this one, overlapping its superior border somewhat. All these strips should be smoothed down and made to adhere firmly to the skin. Applied in this manner, good support will be furnished, and often when the woman arises to the erect position she will remark upon feeling better and stronger at once. It will also help materially in relieving many digestive and nervous symptoms, and be of considerable benefit.

In addition to wearing an elastic or adhesive bandage, attention should be given to the diet, prescribing one suited to the individual, according to the methods outlined in previous chapters. Patients should be enjoined from engaging in physical work of a strenuous character, or in mental activities that are depressing. Symptoms should be treated by their individualization, and the selection of remedies accordingly. Usually the remedies will be those which assist in improving strength and nutrition such as arsenicum, ferrum, calcarea carbonicum, pulsatilla, kali phosphoricum, picric acid, ignatia, sepia, argentum nitricum and many others, the uses of which, and their indications have been freely discussed in the previous chapters of this book.

INDEX